THE
OMEGA-3
CONNECTION

The Groundbreaking Omega-3 Antidepression Diet and Brain Program

∽

ANDREW L. STOLL, M.D.

Simon & Schuster
NEW YORK LONDON TORONTO SYDNEY SINGAPORE

Simon & Schuster
Rockefeller Center
1230 Avenue of the Americas
New York, NY 10020

Copyright © 2001 by Andrew L. Stoll, M.D.

SIMON & SCHUSTER and colophon are registered trademarks
of Simon & Schuster, Inc.
Designed by Stratford Publishing
Manufactured in the United States of America

1   3   5   7   9   10   8   6   4   2

This book contains many details concerning omega-3 fatty acids and other treatments for various medical and psychiatric disorders. Great care was taken to ensure the accuracy of the information in the text. This book is intended to provide general information only, and is not a substitute for medical or psychiatric evaluation and treatment. The author and the publisher are not engaged in providing professional services or medical advice to the individual reader. Each individual's health is unique. All matters regarding health or a particular health situation should be supervised by a health care professional. The author and the publisher shall not be held responsible or liable for any harm or loss allegedly arising, directly or indirectly, from any information in the book.

Copyrighted material used in this book is acknowledged following the index.

Library of Congress Cataloging-in-Publication Data
Stoll, Andrew L. (Andrew Lawrence)
    The omega-3 connection : the groundbreaking omega-3 antidepression diet and brain program / Andrew L. Stoll.
        p.   cm.
Includes bibliographical references and index.
    1. Depression, Mental—Treatment.   2. Manic-depressive illness—Treatment.   3. Omega-3 fatty acids—Therapeutic use.   4. Omega-3 fatty acids—Health aspects.   I. Title.
RC537.S76   2001
616.85'2706—dc21   00-061878
                        ISBN 0-684-87138-6

Acknowledgments

༄ This book would not have been possible without the generous help of many people. I have the utmost gratitude to my patients for their trust in working with me and in creating a partnership to understand and treat their illnesses. My patients have been the best teachers and have always been the inspiration for my research. I would also like to thank Roz Siegel and Andrea Au from Simon & Schuster, who after hearing about my work had the idea for the book, and who kept the momentum going during the long months of researching and writing; Harvard Medical Publications; Pamela Weintraub for her assistance with the manuscript; Maureen Calahan, R.D., for creating the wonderful high omega-3 recipes for the book; Sheldon Roth, M.D., and Cora Roth for their thoughtful comments on the manuscript; Karen Damico and Brian Daly, my research assistants from the Psychopharmacology Research Laboratory at McLean Hospital, who spent hours in the library or on-line tracking down missing facts and figures; Bruce M. Cohen, M.D., Ph.D., head of McLean Hospital, who has always encouraged me to think beyond the bounds of the known facts regarding the brain and behavior; Jonathon F. Borus, M.D., Chief of Psychiatry at Brigham and Women's Hospital, who believed in me enough to encourage me to test the possibility of using fish oil to treat psychiatric disorders; Lauren Marangell, M.D., my friend and Chief of Psychopharmacology at Baylor College of Medicine, who had the faith and courage to be a partner in the omega-3 research; W. Emanuel Severus, M.D., Ph.D., originally from the Free University of Berlin and now working with me at McLean Hospital, who shared that "Eureka!" feeling with me when we discovered the potential of the omega-3 fatty acids in mood disorders; Ross Baldessarini, M.D., Professor of Psychiatry (Neuroscience) at Harvard Medical School and McLean Hospital, one of my early teachers, who along with Dr. Cohen hired me twenty years ago as a college student to work in their lab; Dr. Seth Finkelstein, a neurologist at Massachusetts General Hospital and Harvard Medical School, who taught me the elements of doing clinical and basic research; Dr. Mark Gold, who gave me my first job in psychopharmacology research; Dr. Edmund Fabrizio, my high school organic chemistry teacher, who originally ignited my interest in pharmacology and the scientific method; Doug and Lillian Kelley; my parents, Sondra and Lewis Stoll, who footed the bill for my medical education and did so much more.

I wish to thank my colleagues, friends, and mentors for their support of our studies and helpful advice over the years: Frank Ayd, M.D. (Baltimore, MD); Jonathon O. Cole, M.D. (McLean Hospital and Harvard Medical School); Jerry Cott, Ph.D. (National Institute of Mental Health); Joseph Coyle, M.D. (McLean Hospital and Harvard Medical School); Joseph Hibbeln, M.D. (National Institute of Alcohol Abuse and Alcoholism); David Horrobin, M.D. (Laxdale, Ltd., U.K.); James Hudson, M.D. (McLean Hospital and Harvard Medical School); Robert Katz, Ph.D. (President of the Omega-3 Research Institute, Bethesda, MD); Drs. Paul Keck and Susan McElroy (formerly at McLean Hospital, now at the University of Cincinnati); Alexander Leaf, M.D. (Massachusetts General Hospital and Harvard Medical School); Lawrence Lifson, M.D. (Massachusetts Mental Health Center and Harvard Medical School); Harrison (Skip) Pope, M.D. (McLean Hospital and Harvard Medical School); Bjørn Rene (Pronova Biocare a.s.); Perry F. Renshaw, M.D., Ph.D. (McLean Hospital and Harvard Medical School); Jerrold Rosenbaum, M.D. (Massachusetts General Hospital and Harvard Medical School); Gary Sachs, M.D. (Massachusetts General Hospital and Harvard Medical School); Norman Salem, Ph.D. (National Institute of Alcohol Abuse and Alcoholism); Carl Salzman, M.D. (Massachusetts Mental Health Center, Harvard

Medical School); Artemis P. Simopoulos, M.D. (The Center for Genetics, Nutrition, and Health, Washington, D.C.); Mauricio Tohen, M.D., Dr.P.H. (formerly at McLean Hospital, now at Eli Lilly and Company, Indianapolis, IN); and George Vaillant, M.D. (Brigham and Women's Hospital and Harvard Medical School).

Science cannot proceed without grants, and the following individuals, families, foundations, and agencies made the research possible: The National Alliance for Research in Schizophrenia and Depression (NARSAD), The Hirschhorn Foundation, the Poitras Fund, The Stanley Foundation, The Corporate Alliance for Integrative Medicine Research Program at Harvard Medical School, the National Institute of Mental Health (NIMH), and the National Center for Complementary and Alternative Medicine (NCCAM) of the National Institutes of Health.

My children, Jason, Sarah, and Rebecca, who put up with the endless nights of writing this book, deserve special appreciation. But the most gratitude and appreciation goes to Carol A. Locke, M.D., my wife, whose continuous support made this book possible, and who actually enjoyed the endless hours of researching and discussing the science and the promise of omega-3 fatty acids.

For Carol, Jason, Sarah, and Rebecca,
with boundless love

Contents

Part II
The Omega-3 Renewal Plan

Introduction

༄ For twenty-three years, the swings of bipolar disorder wreaked havoc for one of my female patients, now a forty-five-year-old woman who worked as a research scientist. Despite her expert knowledge of science and medicine, she was unable to find adequate treatment for her condition, marked by dangerous peaks of mania and dark valleys of depression. Her wild swings, especially manic episodes and uncontrolled bouts of anger, could be quelled by two conventional medications effective against bipolar disorder, or manic depression: lithium and Depakote. But for this patient, the cure was almost as devastating as the disease. Dull and depressed and perpetually overweight, she had trouble focusing on her work, enjoying her life, and maintaining relationships with friends. Anxious for a treatment that might balance her mood swings without the cloud of depression, she was fascinated to hear we were testing a natural therapy based on fish oil at Brigham and Women's Hospital in Boston, Massachusetts. Participating in our controlled, double-blind study, in which neither the doctor nor the patient is told who is receiving the real fish oil or who a placebo (an inert look-alike), she nevertheless insisted she "knew" just two weeks into the trial. She knew because not only was her mania gone, but for the first time in decades, the depression had lifted too.

She kept taking fish oil—consisting of fatty acids in the omega-3 category—long after the study was complete. As of this writing, she has been in full remission for three years.

༄ Rome is a wonderful city for culture, but if you're in the throes of mania, you're better off at home. One of my sickest patients suffered his first bout of bipolar disorder in Italy, where he became so manic and disruptive that he wound up in jail. When the police realized he was suffering from a psychiatric disorder, he landed in the locked ward of an Italian hospital. He subsequently escaped, only to endure a second arrest. This time the authorities couldn't wait to get him on an airplane and send him back to the United States. It is a testament to the severity of his symptoms that he was taken from Logan Airport in Boston directly to my office at Brigham and Women's Hospital.

Although conventional treatment based on lithium alone could not act quickly or thoroughly enough for this patient, he did fairly well when we added a powerful antipsychotic medication to the mix. But the side effects were unacceptable, and we were loath to continue the antipsychotic drug for very long. Yet every time he stopped this treatment, his mania returned.

This patient did not want to enter our research study. However, based on my theory that omega-3 fatty acids found in fish oil could help bipolar disorder, he began to eat salmon—a lot of it—at least four ounces a day. It clearly helped, but who can eat that much salmon? He could not keep it up, and without the fish, the symptoms returned.

Fortunately for this patient, we found an answer in fish oil supplements delivering concentrated doses of omega-3 fatty acids including EPA, or eicosapentanoic acid, which circulates in the blood producing powerful hormones and DHA, or docosahexanoic acid, an important component of cell membranes. By adding fish oil to his lithium therapy, this patient was able to keep his mania at bay without resorting to harsh and risky antipsychotic drugs. Today his bipolar illness is in remission, without the burden of medication side effects.

⌒ Suffering severe, untreated bipolar disorder, this next patient was subject to violent rages and crime sprees. Although dynamic and articulate when well, he had already been to prison as a consequence of his illness. Without any relief from the spectrum of available mood-stabilizing drugs, he had one of the most treatment-resistant cases of bipolar disorder I had ever seen.

When given the opportunity to participate in our fish oil study, he was eager indeed. The fish oil was a charm. Participating in our double-blind study, he had no way of knowing whether his capsules contained fish oil or placebo, yet he announced almost immediately that whatever we were giving him, it worked! His mood swings and rages stopped abruptly, and he felt well for the first time in his life. He has remained on fish oil supplements for three years.

∽ These uplifting stories reveal a behind-the-scenes look at my recent study of omega-3 fatty acids and bipolar disorder, published in The Archives of General Psychiatry in May 1999. More powerful than these anecdotes to the research scientists, however, are the data. They show that a group of safe and essential natural oils—the omega-3 fatty acids—have therapeutic value in the treatment of bipolar disorder.

Even more extraordinary perhaps are the emerging findings that omega-3 fatty acids are useful not just in bipolar illness, but perhaps also in depression, postpartum depression, attention deficit–hyperactivity disorder, perhaps stress, and even schizophrenia and autism—in other words, a whole spectrum of psychiatric disease. Because the omega-3 oils are a major constituent of brain cell membranes and are converted to crucial brain chemicals, they are needed for normal nervous system function and seem to be involved in mood regulation, attention and memory, and psychosis. Future studies may link omega-3 deficiency to eating and anxiety disorders as well. In fact, because these oils are essential for the efficient function of every cell in the body, there is established and emerging evidence of therapeutic benefit for the treatment of heart disease, arthritis, diabetes, autoimmune disease, and perhaps even cancer.

The seeming ability of the omega-3s to serve as global brain and body healers reveals not some magical quality, but how incredibly essential the omega-3s are as a foundation for our health and well-being. Deficient, we develop numerous disease states. Repleted, our bodies move to wellness. The clinical and healing power of the omega-3s are backed by hundreds of research studies in well-regarded scientific journals. Taken altogether, these studies establish that our species evolved with a much higher dietary consumption of omega-3 fatty acids than we receive today. These studies have proven oils from fish are safe to consume, even in large dosages and even for the very young and very old. These is no question that omega-3 fatty acid deficiency is widespread in the United States and much of the rest of the developed world, and that we need adequate amounts of this nutrient for optimal health from the moment of conception on. The research shows that omega-3 deficits can lead to a range of mental and physical disorders and that replacement of the missing nutrient may often effect a cure or an amelioration of symptoms.

As you read *The Omega-3 Connection* and its informational guide, the Omega-3 Renewal Plan, you will come to understand the pivotal role omega-3 fatty acids play in physical and mental health. If you live in the United States or anywhere else in the developed world, you can be at risk for omega-3 fatty acid deficiency and all the health problems that entails. In the pages that follow, you will learn how to overcome this sometimes devastating deficit. By following the road map I provide, the Omega-3 Renewal Plan, you can maintain appropriate levels of omega-3, which research suggests can help protect you against many of the most devastating illnesses of our time: heart disease, arthritis, and other major physical problems, as well as depression, bipolar disorder, attention deficit–hyperactivity disorder, and other forms of psychiatric disease.

Part I

THE OMEGA-3 DEFICIT

1

Nature's Mood Enhancers

➣ During the course of reading this book you will learn about exciting research into a remarkable group of natural substances: the omega-3 fatty acids. Omega-3 fatty acids are essential for the optimal function of every cell in our bodies, yet we cannot manufacture them internally. Instead, along with vitamins, these essential oils can be obtained only in the diet.

Over the past century, people in developed countries, particularly in the United States, have largely eliminated omega-3 fatty acids from their diet. There is considerable evidence that this has had a very negative impact on the inner workings of many bodily systems, most notably the heart and the brain. We are learning that restoring the body's natural balance of omega-3 oils may improve a multitude of medical disorders, including coronary artery disease, major depression, and bipolar disorder (also called manic-depressive illness). My personal journey toward discovery of the omega-3 oils began in 1987, when I finished medical school and launched my career in psychiatric neuroscience with a residency and fellowship at Harvard Medical School and McLean Hospital in Belmont, Massachusetts. The focus of my clinical work and research was (and still is) bipolar disorder, one of the most complex, dangerous, and fascinating medical disorders—and one of just a handful of afflictions that occur only in humans.

The prevalence of bipolar disorder suggests that it is not merely some random unlucky mutation, but that the genes involved might have been preferentially selected during the evolution of the human species. Without bipolar illness, our species would, at best, be uninteresting, even boring; at worst, the human race might not have survived the challenges of our evolutionary and society history at all.

Why would such a life-threatening disorder be necessary for our species? Viewed through the lens of history, some people believe its evolutionary value is clear. Kay Redfield Jamison, professor of psychiatry at Johns Hopkins University, has written extensively on the creative and leadership qualities of the many people throughout history who have been retrospectively diagnosed with bipolar disorder. From Winston Churchill and Ted Turner to Vincent van Gogh, Georgia O'Keefe, Virginia Woolf, and Charles Mingus, some of the volatile, grandiose individuals with this affliction have launched and dismantled empires, revolutionized cultures, and rendered hauntingly beautiful works of art. Bipolar disorder, characterized by alternating cycles of melancholy and mania, is especially prevalent among those in leadership and creative fields. A long list of writers, artists, and musicians—Ernest Hemingway, Michelangelo, and Cole Porter, to name a few—have produced visionary work, despite the crests and valleys of their mood states. According to Jamison, many prominent poets of our century have suffered from bipolar disorder, including Sylvia Plath and Hart Crane, and in the years before the advent of effective treatments, many killed themselves.

The occurrence of bipolar disorder is not limited to the arts. It is highly prevalent in the computer, biotechnology, and high finance fields, where some of the most creative and globally transforming work is currently being done.

Most people with bipolar disorder, of course, are not celebrities, but the wide swings between highs and lows disrupt their lives just as much, devastating relationships, school, jobs, and quality of life. Between 10 percent and 20 percent of bipolar patients will die of their illness, usually through suicide.

My career as a psychiatrist has been dedicated to relief and prevention of pain and suffering from these mood disorders. As a physician-neuroscientist, understanding and treating bipolar disorder has provided me with a profound yet still embryonic view of the biochemistry of the brain. In medical school, I was taught that if you can understand diabetes, you will understand all of medicine because those with diabetes fall prey to many other disorders, from cardiac disease to kidney failure to stroke. Similarly, if you understand bipolar disorder, you will have special insight into psychiatry because those with bipolar disorder manifest a wide variety of psychiatric symptoms. In the full-blown disorder, periods of suicidal depression alternate with episodes of mania: euphoria, irritability, increased energy, decreased need for sleep, and racing thoughts accompanied by impulsive behaviors and grandiose ideas. Symptoms of anxiety and even psychosis may occur during different phases of the illness.

As devastating as bipolar disorder can be, it is treatable with drugs. But working with patients who have bipolar illness at McLean and Brigham and Women's Hospitals, I sometimes found the standard pharmaceutical agents ineffective or so harsh that they produced temporary discomfort or caused permanent medical problems of their own. Ongoing psychiatric symptoms, serious side effects, and noncompliance with medication therapy were the frequent results. These outcomes are even more pronounced in teaching hospitals like McLean and Brigham and Women's, where many of the patients have more severe or treatment-resistant conditions.

The long-term treatment of patients with bipolar disorder relies on the so-called mood stabilizers such as lithium and valproate. These often produce dramatically good results long term and have saved thousands of lives. Unfortunately, patients using lithium often experience weight gain, tremors, increased urination, drowsiness, and acne. Some 15 percent suffer reduced thyroid function, and as many as 5 percent develop kidney problems. Often the biggest problem for these innately creative individuals on lithium can be a loss of the creative spark. While their manias are under control, their emotions are frequently flattened, and they are, to use a clinical term, "cognitively dulled." What is more, one mood stabilizer used alone is often not effective over the long term. In an effort to control recurrent manias or depressions, patients might end up taking two or more mood stabilizers at once, increasing their risk of side effects and drug interactions.

As a psychopharmacologist (a psychiatrist specializing in medication treatments) and researcher with responsibility for treating these desperately ill people, my mandate was clear: to find newer medications with fewer side effects that worked as well as or better than the ones already in use, and to increase our understanding of the disorder.

Working with the German researcher W. Emanuel Severus, M.D., I started the hunt for a better treatment in 1993. Our strategy was to conduct extensive computer searches of medical research papers to identify substances whose biochemical properties were similar to the standard mood stabilizers, lithium and valproate. Reviewing hundreds of papers in search of a candidate molecule (one that had never been used in psychiatric disorders), we pulled up one match time and again: omega-3 fatty acids, or common fish oil!

At first our reaction was surprise and disbelief. We had no evidence that omega-3 fatty acids would be helpful in bipolar disorder, yet it made sense. Already used by some physicians in the treatment of heart disease, Crohn's disease, and rheumatoid arthritis, these oils are precursors to important signaling molecules in the body and are essential components of the healthy cell membrane—the same membranes that appear to mediate the activity of lithium and valproate in the brain. The omega-3 fatty acids are found in unusually high concentration in the brain. Although almost nothing in the literature connected them with bipolar disorder, the possibility that they might act to stabilize mood was very real.

Our subsequent clinical study, ultimately published in *The Archives of General Psychiatry*, suggested that these safe and natural oils had therapeutic value in the treatment of bipolar disorder. In this one study, looking at thirty patients over four months, omega-3 fatty acids, used alone or with other medications, enabled a few seemingly incurable patients to lead normal lives and enhanced mood stability for those already gaining some benefit from other medications. Omega-3 fatty acids were also safer than valproate and lithium: they had few side effects, and, in my practice, at least, they have become one of the most frequently used "medications" for patients with mood disorders.

But there is more. While our discovery emerged from a search for a new treatment of bipolar disorder, evidence points to far wider applications for omega-3 fatty acids in the care and nurturing of the brain. Studies now under way indicate considerable potential as an antidepressant in the more common type of mood disorder, termed unipolar major depression. Other research suggests that omega-3 fatty acids may yield new treatments for postpartum depression, schizophrenia, attention deficit–hyperactivity disorder, and possibly many other disorders as well. They may be very appropriate for children and the elderly, whose bodies often cannot tolerate conventional psychiatric medications. Furthermore, it is possible that omega-3 fatty acids may actually prevent these disorders from developing at all.

For those of us engaging in neuroscience research, the possibility of global healing power for this natural lipid makes sense. Until the twentieth century, omega-3 fatty acids, derived largely from cold water oily fish from the ocean or freshwater lakes and rivers, as well as wild animals and plants, were common elements of the human diet. Today, with the advent of processed foods and the reduction of omega-3 fatty acids in the typical Western diet, that has changed.

We often think of depression and bipolar disorder as purely hereditary in nature, but research on the omega-3 fatty acids indicates that some of what is inherited may not be in the genes. In studies of omega-3–deprived mice, scientists learned that it may take several generations for offspring to deplete their brains of omega-3 fatty acids. This is because the body tenaciously holds on to the omega-3s throughout life, and also because most of the omega-3s in young animals come from what their mother (and her mother) have consumed and stored. Over time, of course, depletion occurs. Could this possibly be one reason that depression and other mood disorders are on the rise in the United States, or be a factor in the apparently low rate of depression in Japan and other countries where the consumption of fish has remained high for generations?

Researchers in psychiatric epidemiology have found that the prevalence of depression varies as much as sixty-fold from country to country. In a fascinating study from Joseph Hibbeln, M.D., of the National Institute on Alcohol Abuse and Alcoholism, data shows that the international pattern of major depression corresponds strongly to cross-national differences in coronary artery disease, suggesting similar dietary risk factors. Of all the dietary variables, fish consumption appears to be the most significant, with fish-eating nations at lower risk for both major depression and heart disease.

There is evidence that omega-3 deficiency may play a role in postpartum depression as well. The developing fetus and newborn require high amounts of omega-3 fatty acids and receive them through the placenta and breast milk, respectively. The baby's ability to import and incorporate omega-3 oils outweighs the typical Western mother's ability to replace what she has lost. It is well-documented that infants and toddlers who were breast fed rather than bottle fed score higher on cognitive and visual system tests. It has been determined that one reason is the high levels of long-chain omega-3 fatty acids in breast milk. (There are none in U.S. formula.) If the mother does not maintain sufficient levels of omega-3 fatty acids in her diet, she puts her body at risk of depletion during the pregnancy and breast-feeding period. Low levels of omega-3 in her brain and body may put her at greater risk for depression and possibly other disorders.

In studies of children with attention deficit–hyperactivity disorder (ADHD), meanwhile, Jay R. Burgess of Purdue University has found that some 40 percent showed evidence of omega-3 fatty acid deficiency. Research into use of omega-3 supplements as an adjunctive treatment for ADHD is currently under way.

Although the results of the ADHD studies are not yet in, research with healthy populations indicate that omega-3 fatty acids may indeed play a role in attention as well as cognitive abilities like memory and response time. In a fifty-day study of 285 normal women, with a particular focus on EPA, David Benton, Ph.D., a researcher at the University of Wales Swansea, found that omega-3 fatty acid supplements improved measurements of memory, vigilance, and mood.

The jury will remain out on many of these treatments and applications until controlled clinical studies are completed and replicated. In the meantime if you are already receiving drug therapy for a psychiatric disorder and would like to start taking omega-3 fatty acids, it is important that you continue current treatment and consult with your clinician. In most cases, the omega-3 fatty acids are used "adjunctively"; that is, added to what you already take. There are some patients with mood disorders doing very well on omega-3 fatty acids alone but until more data are in, I do not recommend treatment based solely on omega-3 fatty acid therapy, except for the mildest forms of depression or bipolar disorder, or for the general population, to enhance well-being, mood, and health. If you think you might have a mood disorder, you should consult a mental health care professional to review your treatment options.

The chapters that follow present the latest findings on omega-3 fatty acids and mood enhancement—not just for those who suffer from bipolar disorder, but possibly for everyone. And because the use of this supplement in psychiatry is so new, I'll deliver a road map for use in my Omega-3 Renewal Plan. What foods are especially rich in omega-3 fatty acids, and how much should you eat? What should you look for in a supplement? What can labels tell you? How much should you take and when?

I understand that some readers may be skeptical. Who is to say this is not just another supplement flavor of the month, another bogus claim in the continual stream of magic elixirs and miracle cures? Who is to say that fish oil is not really snake oil, a fad that will pass as others have before? Well, it may. The case we present to you is not yet solid. Many more studies are needed. But serious scientists at many prestigious institutions like Harvard Medical School, Oregon Health Sciences University, Purdue University, the University Hospital of Ghent in Belgium, and the University of Sheffield in the United Kingdom are impressed enough to be dedicating themselves to the study of the omega-3 fatty acids.

Every so often, scientists really do discover a substance of transformative power, one with the ability to cure the previously incurable and improve the quality of life for the rest of us. Omega-3 fatty acids—a component of simple fish oil, once so prevalent in our diet but now largely absent—could be such a substance.

2

The Fat of Life:
A Nutritional Guide to Fatty Acids

෴ One of the great medical myths of the past fifty years has been the notion that fats (more properly called lipids) are evil. Of course, like all other enduring myths, there is a grain of truth at the core. Literally thousands of studies over the past half century have traced high-fat diets to increased risk of heart disease. The most famous of these, the Framingham Heart Study, followed a representative sample of 5,209 adults in Framingham, Massachusetts, to examine the circumstances and risk factors associated with heart disease. The Framingham study was an epidemiological study designed to learn how those who develop cardiovascular diseases differed from those who remain free of the diseases over a long period of time. Epidemiology is a branch of medical science devoted to the large-scale study of populations and disease; epidemiologists search for risk factors and causes of illnesses through statistical associations and other methods.

Along with such culprits as smoking and sedentary lifestyle, the Framingham scientists found danger in diets high in fat. This study and many others over the past few decades have driven the point home: diets high in fatty foods, from bacon to butter to red meat, greatly increase our chances of acquiring cardiovascular disease, reducing not just the length but also the quality of life. The problem is not simply excessive amounts of fat or cholesterol clogging arteries or adding inches to our waistlines. Certain fats, like the omega-6 and omega-3 fatty acids act as powerful hormone-like agents, playing many roles in health and disease. The Framingham scientists, with their focus on cholesterol and saturated fats, overlooked the damaging effects of another type of fat, the omega-6 fats.

With a genuine paradigm shift, we must develop an accurate view of the diversity of fats, with a range of health benefits and risks. Although some dietary fats are implicated in heart disease, others may reduce the risk of these illnesses, and even treat or prevent a range of other diseases, such as arthritis, depression, and diabetes. Some lipids suppress inflammation, others promote it. Some fats raise cholesterol, others lower it. Some make cell membranes rigid, others render them flexible.

The Essential Fats

The data from the medical literature are clear: do not lump all types of dietary fat together in a single, negative category. Excessive consumption of saturated fat and cholesterol certainly can cause disease and a greater chance of early death. But other fats, termed the essential fats, are necessary for optimal health. In the yin and yang of proper physiological balance, the essential fatty acids—the omega-3 and omega-6 oils—are health enhancers.

I want to stop here to point out my use of the term oil. We have used the term fat in a general way, but oils and fats (both lipids) differ in their chemical structures. Oils (olive, canola, and fish oil, for instance) are liquid at room temperature; fats (butter and lard) are solid. These subtle chemical differences produce vastly different chemical effects in the body.

The role of the essential fatty acids in the body and brain can be best understood in terms of what we know about lipids—fats as well as oils—and their impact on health and disease.

The Cholesterol Issue

Researchers investigating risk factors in the Framingham study initially homed in on not so much the total consumption of lipids, but on detection of high blood levels of one particular lipid: cholesterol. A soft, waxy substance found among other lipids in the bloodstream and in the body's cells, cholesterol is needed to form cell membranes, certain hormones, and specific tissues.

Like other lipids, cholesterol cannot dissolve in the bloodstream, which is mostly water, and must be transported throughout the body by carriers in the blood called lipoproteins. Two lipoproteins are particularly important. The low-density lipoproteins (LDLs), when carrying cholesterol, are sometimes called "bad" cholesterol, and high-density lipoproteins (HDLs) are also known as "good" cholesterol when combined with cholesterol.

Too much LDL cholesterol circulating in the blood within a pro-inflammatory environment can promote atherosclerosis ("hardening of the arteries"), which is the buildup of a thick, hard coating called plaque within the walls of the arteries. Just like a clogged pipe, if arterial walls accumulate too much plaque, blood flowing through them will be blocked. Arterial plaque can block flow of blood to the heart, leading to heart attack (myocardial infarction), or block the flow of blood to the brain, causing a stroke (cerebrovascular accident).

About a quarter of all cholesterol is carried through the body by HDLs, thought to be beneficial. The data suggesting that HDLs promote health come from two sources: epidemiological studies linking high levels of HDL to lower rates of heart disease and laboratory studies examining exactly what HDL does to cholesterol at a cellular or molecular level. The latest studies indicate that HDL's role is complex, but that one of its actions is to carry cholesterol away from the arteries and back to the liver, where it is passed from the body. Some experts believe that HDL cholesterol can even break down the cholesterol in plaque, potentially leading to a reopening of partially clogged arteries.

According to the American Heart Association, excess cholesterol in the body comes from two sources: (1) the liver, which produces about 1,000 milligrams of cholesterol a day from other substances; (2) dietary saturated fat and cholesterol of the sort that are found in animals and dairy products.

Grouping the Fatty Acids: Essential and Nonessential Fats

Researchers today realize that not all fats are created equal. Anyone who does supermarket shopping is likely to know there are four major categories of fat listed in the labels of the foods we eat: cholesterol, saturated fatty acids, monounsaturated fatty acids, and polyunsaturated fatty acids. Of the three fatty acid categories, only one—the saturated fats found in animal and dairy products—have been implicated in raising LDL, or bad cholesterol. Most foods contain a combination of all three fatty acids in differing proportions. Nutritionists assign foods to a general fat category based on the proportions of each fatty acid contained in the product (see Table 2–1).

What You See Is What You Get: Fatty Acids Function Based on Their Chemical Form

Like other biochemicals, fatty acids function based on their chemical structure. Essentially chains of carbon atoms with hydrogen atoms attached off to the side, the various fatty acids differ based on the number of carbon atoms in the chain and the types of bonds they share with each other (see Figure 2–1).

Fat in 3D: The Chemical Structure of the Fatty Acids

In essence, chemical bonds are created when electrons are shared between two atoms. This sharing of electrons makes atoms stick together (a bond). Carbon atoms found in nature always have four bonds available to link up with other atoms. Since the carbons are in a chain, it makes sense that two of those bonds are usually taken up with links to adjacent carbon atoms. That leaves two bonds open for other atoms, usually hydrogen. If two hydrogen atoms attach to each carbon atom in the chain, that chain is said to be "saturated"—it contains as much hydrogen as possible, with each carbon-carbon bond consisting of a single, shared electron.

Saturated fatty acids are very stable chemicals. They are also solid or stiff at room temperature. In fact, the processed foods industry uses so much saturated fat precisely because of its chemical stability and solid, pliable form.

When fatty acids are "unsaturated," it means that some of the carbon atoms in the chain have double bonds with each other and less hydrogen is present—hence the term unsaturated. The carbon-carbon double bond is the chemical signature of an unsaturated fat. Monounsaturated fats have a single double bond, and polyunsaturated fats have two or more.

Solid, Liquid, and in-Between

The differing chemical structures of the fatty acids lead to a useful variety of attributes in the physical world. The saturated fatty acids are generally solid in form, like butter, even at room temperature, and are the most chemically stable. Most of the time we consume saturated fatty acids in meat, dairy, and processed food products, including beef, veal, lamb, pork, lard, poultry, butter, cream, milk, cheese, cookies, and crackers.

Coconut and palm oil (known as the tropical oils) contain a

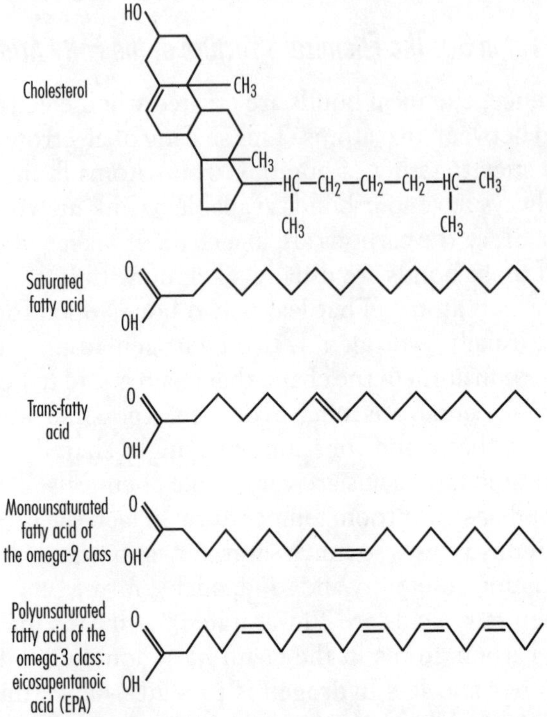

FIGURE 2–1: Chemical Structures of Cholesterol and Examples of Saturated, Trans-, Monounsaturated, and Polyunsaturated Fatty Acids

Note the large difference in the chemical structures between cholesterol (a sterol) and the fatty acids. Among the four fatty acids in the figure, the superficial similarity of the chemical structures is misleading because the presence of carbon-carbon double bonds (denoted by the double lines in the chemical structures) gives rise to fatty acids with vastly different biochemical properties in the body. For example, only the polyunsaturated fatty acids (omega-3 and omega-6 fatty acids), with their multiple double bonds are converted into crucial signaling molecules in the body and brain, known as eicosanoids (prostaglandins are one example of an eicosanoid). There are other consequences of multiple double bonds in the chemical structure of a fat. Every double bond produces a separate "kink" in the carbon chain, leading to many potential three-dimensional configurations, which leads to greater mobility of the polyunsaturated molecule. It is this enhanced mobility that keeps polyunsaturated fats liquid at room temperature and which may produce healthy, fluid cell membranes at body temperature. The greater membrane fluidity or possibly some other effect of the polyunsaturated fatty acids alters the function of neurotransmitter receptors and other important signaling proteins embedded in the cell membrane.

TABLE 2–1: Lipid Composition of Various Plant Oils and Animal Fats

The lipids (fats and oils) in most foods are a mixture comprised of all three fatty acid categories as well as cholesterol in various proportions. This table shows the fatty acid and cholesterol content of various dietary oils and fats.

Oil or Fat	Cholesterol (mg)	Saturated gram %	Monounsaturated gram %	Polyunsaturated gram %	Polyunsaturated gram % (omega-3)[a]		
					C18	C20	C22
Beef tallow	109	48.4	40.5	3.1	0.6	0	0
Black currant seed oil	0	0	12.4	62.8[b]	15.4	0	0
Borage seed (starflower) oil	0	15	19	57.4[b]	0	0	0
Butter fat	256	61.9	28.7	3.7	1.5	0	0
Canola (rapeseed) oil	0	6.8	55.5	33.3	11.1	0	0
Coconut oil	0	86.5	5.8	1.8	0	0	0
Corn oil	0	12.7	24.2	58.0	0.7	0	0
Cottonseed oil	0	25.8	17.8	51.5	0.2	0	0
Evening primrose oil	0	—	8.0	78[b]	0.2	0	0
Flaxseed (linseed) oil	0	9.4	20.2	66.0	53.3	0	0
Lard	95	39.2	45.1	11.2	1.0	0	0
Olive oil	0	13.2	73.6	7.9	0.6	0	0
Palm oil	0	48.9	37.0	9.1	0.2	0	0
Peanut oil	0	11.8	46.1	32.0	0	0	0
Safflower oil	0	6.8	18.6	70.1	0	0	0
Salmon oil	485	23.8	39.7	29.9	1.0	8.8	11.1
Sesame oil	0	14.2	45.4	40.4	0	0	0
Soybean oil	0	14.4	23.3	57.9	6.8	0	0
Sunflower oil	0	8.7	25.1	66.2	0	0	0
Walnut oil	0	9.1	22.8	63.3	10.4	0	0

[a] The omega-3 fatty acids, C18=alpha-linolenic acid (ALA); C20=eicosapentanoic acid (EPA); C22 = docosahexanoic acid (DHA).

[b] Black currant seed oil, borage seed oil, and evening primrose oil contain high concentrations of gamma-linolenic acid (GLA), an omega-6 fatty acid with less inflammatory properties than other omega-6 fatty acids.

Sources: Handbook of Chemistry and Physics, 74th ed. (Cleveland, Ohio: CRC Press, 1998); Health Effects of Polyunsaturated Fatty Acids in Seafoods, A. P. Simopoulos, R. R. Kifer, R. E. Martin, eds. (Orlando, FL: Academic Press, 1986); Dietary Fats and Health, E. G. Perkins and W. J. Visek, eds. (American Oil Chemists' Society, 1983). The sources of the fatty acid content of black currant oil, borage seed oil, and evening primrose oil are from selected manufacturers' Web sites.

high proportion of saturated fatty acids. Because of their specific fatty acid composition, the tropical oils are liquids at room temperature. The tropical oils are used widely in food processing because, as liquids, they are easy to handle, and because of their saturated fat content, they extend the shelf life of many foods. While useful to the food industry, however, these fats and oils can contribute to coronary artery disease.

Also hazardous to health are the so-called trans-fatty acids, found in margarine and other synthetic foods. Created in the laboratory, trans-fatty acids result when manufacturers add hydrogen to unsaturated vegetable oil. Due to the configuration of the new chemical bonds—different from those found in most naturally occurring saturated fatty acids—trans-fatty acids are even more stable than those of saturated fatty acids. The advantage is longer shelf life without spoiling for processed foods. The disadvantages, according to a spate of recent studies, include risk for coronary heart disease in excess of that associated with saturated fat.

The American Heart Association (AHA) has put its stamp of approval on unsaturated fatty acids in both monounsaturated and polyunsaturated categories as healthier substitutes for saturated fats. Generally liquid at room temperature but prone to solidify when refrigerated, oils containing high amounts of monounsaturated lipids derive from canola, olives, peanuts, and avocados. Oils containing high amounts of polyunsaturated lipids—found in safflower oil, fish oil, flax, and sunflower seeds, among numerous other sources—remain as liquids, whether refrigerated or not.

Referring to extensive scientific evidence, the AHA literature today emphatically states that monounsaturated and polyunsaturated fatty acids may not only be healthier than saturated fatty acids, but may actually reverse the latter's devastating effects. By increasing the body's supply of HDL cholesterol, monounsaturated and polyunsaturated fatty acids can keep blood cholesterol levels down and reduce cholesterol deposits in artery walls. The problem is that the Framingham Study and the AHA do not differentiate between the two major types of polyunsaturated fatty acids: omega-3 and omega-6. A diet based on vegetable oil (high in omega-6) will produce a vastly different state of health than one balanced with omega-3 oils.

The AHA also strongly recommends a low-fat diet, with no more than 30 percent of calories from fat of any sort. The reasoning is rooted in the findings of the Framingham Heart Study. With obesity a major risk factor for heart disease, it makes sense to limit calories, no matter how beneficial the source. And fat of any sort is calorie-rich.

The Fat Wars

Representing the mainstream, the AHA is not the only game in town. One alternative approach, pioneered by California heart researcher Dr. Dean Ornish, calls for intensive daily exercise and a diet allowing no more than 10 percent of the daily calories to come from fat. Studies show that the Ornish approach can actually reverse the ravages of heart disease without drugs or surgery. In practice, however, many people might find it difficult to adhere to such a rigorous program over the long term.

Taking an opposite tack, others argue for diets high in fat. The best-known figure promoting a high-fat diet for weight loss is Dr. Robert C. Atkins, whose best-selling *Dr. Atkins' New Diet Revolution* argues that carbohydrates, not fat, are the true villains in the battle of the bulge. The Atkins diet permits as much fat as desired as long as carbohydrates are kept at bay. The diet can lead to marked weight loss, but without motivation, it is difficult to maintain. In addition, the long-term health consequences (if any) of this "unnatural" proportion of fat to carbohydrate is unknown.

The Mediterranean Diet

Yet others, such as physician and nutrition scientist Artemis Simopoulos, M.D., advocate the Mediterranean Diet, based on the eating habits of Mediterranean regions like southern Italy, Greece, and Crete. The Mediterranean diet includes staples of fruits, vegetables, and grains, drawing as well some 30 percent of its calories from olive oil and other mono- and polyunsaturated fats.

The first inkling that the Mediterranean diet might bolster health came in the 1970s, when Dr. Ancel Keys and colleagues at the University of Minnesota examined the relationship between diet and heart disease in seven countries. They found that those who lived by the Mediterranean Sea suffered a fraction of the heart disease found in the United States and other Western nations. Keys noted that Mediterranean populations consumed dietary fat largely derived from fish and vegetables, as opposed to the highly saturated animal and dairy fats typical of the West.

The subject of intense debate, Keys's findings have nonetheless been confirmed in numerous prominent studies over the past ten years. Most notable is the recent research conducted by Dr. Michel de Lorgeril and colleagues in Lyon, France. In that study, 30 percent of the calories in the experimental Mediterranean diet came from fat, but only 8 percent from saturated fat. In a control group, 34 percent of the calories were from fat, with almost 12 percent from saturated fat. Lorgeril observed that the group on the Mediterranean diet had far lower rates of cardiac disease. And in a boon for the omega-3 fatty acid camp, participants with the highest blood levels of omega-3 fatty acids were at lowest risk of all.

Essential Fatty Acids and the New Fat Paradigm

In the midst of all this brouhaha, a new series of studies has quietly reframed the high-fat/low-fat debate. Although not yet extensively covered in the popular press, the latest research shows that polyunsaturated fatty acids, long grouped with monounsaturated fatty acids as enemies of cholesterol, are more complex and diverse than previously thought, with many unique and important roles in the body and brain.

Already known to lower the risk of having a heart attack and protecting against sudden death during a heart attack, polyunsaturated fats of the omega-3 class may also be responsible for protecting against arthritis, diabetes, and some psychiatric disorders. The reason is their ability to control many of the most basic functions of the cell. Omega-3 fatty acids are vital nutrients controlling energy production within each cell. They are also converted throughout the body to myriad messenger molecules essential for influencing a host of physiological functions.

The essential fatty acids are also the major building blocks of cellular membranes surrounding every cell in the body. Known as lipid bilayers (because they are made of two layers of fat), cell membranes serve as an effective barrier to unwanted substances and also function as highly selective molecular portals to the inside of each cell. These fatty acid walls help control the opening and closing of the cell's channels to a diversity of compounds, thus influencing the most basic cellular functions.

Like vitamin C, calcium, and a host of other essential nutrients not manufactured by the body, most polyunsaturated acids must be consumed as a regular part of the diet for us to thrive. Most fats, of course, are manufactured by the body, as anyone on a weight-loss program is likely to learn. Eat too much protein or carbohydrate and your body will all too readily convert these nutrients for storage as fat. For many years, nutritionists thought that polyunsaturated fats were created in the body as well. But in 1929, George M. Burr and Mildred M. Burr of the University of Minnesota reported that rats fed a fat-free diet failed to grow, lost weight, developed scaly skin and kidney damage, and died prematurely. These conditions could be prevented and reversed only with the addition of one type of polyunsaturated fat: linoleic acid, an omega-6 oil. At that time, omega-3 fatty acids could not be isolated. Today, it is clear that both omega-6 and omega-3 fatty acids are necessary for optimal health.

This study and others caused nutritionists to group the polyunsaturated fats with the essential nutrients—those required for survival but not produced by the body—and to name them essential fatty acids (EFAs). We now know that EFAs come

The first double bond starts with the third
carbon atom from the end in omega-3 fatty acids.

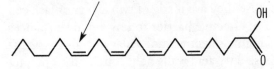

Eicosapentanoic
acid (EPA):
20-carbon omega-3
fatty acid

The first double bond starts with the sixth
carbon atom from the end in omega-6 fatty acids.

Arachidonoic
acid (AA):
20-carbon omega-6
fatty acid

FIGURE 2–2: Chemical Structures of the Omega-3 and Omega-6 Fatty Acids

The omega-3 and omega-6 fatty acids have very similar chemical structures—both are long chain and polyunsaturated. The terms of omega-3 and omega-6 indicate where the first carbon-carbon double bond is located, counting from the end of the carbon chain opposite the acid group. The most amazing feature of the polyunsaturated fatty acids is that the subtle difference in chemical structure between EPA (omega-3) and arachidonic acid (omega-6)—just two hydrogen atoms— produces profound differences in what the omega-3s and omega-6s do in the body. Omega-3 fatty acids are found mostly in oily fish and some uncommon but edible plants. The source of omega-6 fatty acids are most often vegetable and seed oils, which are very common in our diet. The most current data suggest that humans evolved eating a balance of omega-3 and omega-6 fatty acids. There is now a considerable amount of evidence that this shift in our diet away from omega-3s has resulted in higher rates of many medical illnesses, particularly heart disease and depression. In fact, a recent international conference recommended an ideal ratio of omega-6 to omega-3 to be 1 to 1. Contrast that with the prevailing current U.S. ratio of omega-6 to omega-3 of 10 or 20 to 1.

in two basic categories: omega-6 fatty acids and their counter-parts, the omega-3 fatty acids, both named for the position of the first double bond in the carbon chain. As polyunsaturated lipids, both omega-6 and omega-3 fatty acids have multiple double bonds. The first double bond in the omega-6 class begins at the sixth carbon atom from the end of the chain. Omega-3 fatty acids differ in a subtle yet crucial way, in that they have their first double bond at the third carbon position (see Figure 2–2). This one difference—the absence of only two hydrogen atoms—is what makes the omega-3 fatty acids unique and essential for optimal health.

The challenge is getting sufficient quantities of omega-3 fatty acids. In the United States and many other developed countries, the modern food supply is low in omega-3 oils. This omega-3 deficiency, evidence now suggests, may underlie a multitude of health problems in both children and adults. The omega-6 oils are also essential nutrients required for health, but modern diets contain more than enough to meet our needs.

The implications of omega-3 deficiency on the brain are profound and span the entire human life cycle. Beginning in pregnancy, premature birth and its potential neurologic complications may result from omega-3 deficiency. Babies who are bottle-fed or born from omega-3-deficient mothers will lack the omega-3 fatty acids necessary for optimal cognitive and visual development. Children deprived of omega-3s may have less ability to pay attention and control impulsive behavior and may be at higher risk for depression. Teenagers and adults with omega-3 deficiency may be more prone to hostility or violence. In aging, the loss of omega-3 fatty acids in the brain may result in a higher risk of stroke, memory problems, or dementia. Individuals of *any age* without adequate amounts of omega-3 fatty acids in the brain and body may also be at higher risk for depression, bipolar disorder, and possibly other psychiatric disorders.

The Yin and Yang of Fat Science

There is balance in nature, and one example of its elegant expression is the tightly linked biochemistry of the two essential fatty acid groups, the omega-6 and omega-3 oils. Unlike other lipids, neither is made in the human body; rather, these essential fatty acids are synthesized in the chloroplasts of plants. The chloroplast, the green, chlorophyll-containing structure in plant cells, converts sunlight and carbon dioxide into oxygen and a range of complex organic molecules, including sugars, proteins, and lipids. Only chloroplasts within certain plants (e.g., marine and freshwater algae) produce high quantities of long-chain omega-3 fatty acids.

We derive omega-6 fatty acids from a commonly available range of vegetable and seed oils, including corn oil, olive oil, sunflower oil, and safflower oil. The long-chain omega-3 fatty acids are more difficult to obtain through the modern Western diet and most often come indirectly, through the oils of fish that have received omega-3 fatty acids through the food chain, ultimately from omega-3-producing algae and other water-based plants. A shorter-chain omega-3 fatty acid is available in walnuts, flaxseeds, and some other plant sources.

Once in the body, omega-3 and omega-6 fatty acids follow parallel pathways, continually competing with each other for chemical conversion to various structures and molecules inside and outside of cells. Given this mechanism, it makes sense that the two fats might be required in approximately equal amounts. Hoping to reach a consensus on the issue, the National Institutes of Health recently sponsored an international conference for omega-3 researchers across a range of disciplines, from psychiatry and cardiology to nutrition and immunology. It is notable that despite the diversity of their backgrounds, the researchers agreed virtually unanimously: for optimum health, omega-6 and omega-3 fatty acids should be eaten in approximately equal proportions—a ratio of 1 to 1.

This stands in stark contrast to the modern Western diet, where that ratio is often highly skewed to ten to twenty times more omega-6 than omega-3 (a ratio of 10 or 20 to 1). Our dietary imbalance has shifted crucial biochemical pathways toward the more abundant omega-6 fatty acids, leading to negative changes in numerous body systems, possibly including the brain regions contributing to mood. Medical science is only beginning to comprehend the power and complexity of omega-6/omega-3 balance.

Pathways to Health

Once eaten and absorbed by the body, omega-6 and omega-3 fatty acids go through a series of biochemical conversions. This metamorphosis can be divided into two major pathways.

In the first pathway, the omega-6 and omega-3 fatty acids become incorporated into cell membranes. Without access to sufficient quantities of omega-3 and omega-6 fatty acids, cell membranes will incorporate saturated and other types of fat instead. Membrane walls rich in the omega-3 fatty acids will be more fluid because polyunsaturated fats have lower melting points than saturated fats. (Remember that polyunsaturated fats are liquid even at low temperatures.) Among the health benefits that may result from a diet high in omega-3 oils and the ideal fluidity of cell membranes, according to scientific reports, are superior cognition and visual development in babies and lower risk for cardiovascular disease in adults.

In the second pathway, the essential fatty acids are converted to a series of intermediate molecules and then ultimately to hormonelike substances called the eicosanoids, an umbrella term for several classes of cell-signaling molecules, most notably the prostaglandins. The prostaglandins mediate the "inflammatory process," a crucial and finely tuned mechanism that fights infection, heals tissue injury, and performs a multitude of other functions within the immune system, the cardiovascular system, and even the brain.

Omega-6 fatty acids produce strongly inflammatory or "reactive" eicosanoids while omega-3 fatty acids produce less inflammatory or even anti-inflammatory eicosanoids. One can begin to see the profound health implications here. When in balance, essential fatty acids promote optimal health perhaps by their fluidizing effect on cell membranes or by the proportions of various eicosanoid derivatives. When out of balance, they can throw the body into chaos.

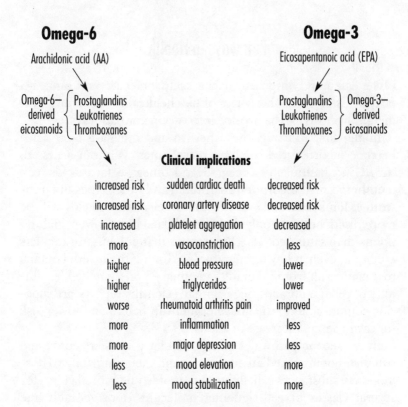

FIGURE 2–3: The Omega-6–Omega-3 Balancing Act

The Essential Difference

Although EFAs are cousins to saturated fatty acids, they live in stark contrast to those rigid, relatively inert molecules. The root of the difference is chemical structure. The carbon chain in saturated fat is straight and rigid, in contrast to the bent, twisting, and flexible structure of the polyunsaturated fatty acids.

Every double bond in an EFA produces a separate kink in the carbon chain, leading to many potential three-dimensional configurations, which leads to greater mobility of the polyunsaturated molecule. It is this enhanced mobility that keeps polyunsaturated fats liquid at room temperature and produces healthy, fluid cell membranes at body temperature.

Ideally, omega-6 fatty acids work in tandem with the omega-3s (see Fig 2–3). When in balance, eicosanoid derivatives of the omega-3 fatty acids keep the omega-6–derived eicosanoids in check. For example, pro-inflammatory eicosanoids (prostaglandins) derived from omega-6 fatty acids enable the immune system to fight serious infection and also set the stage for labor and delivery at the end of pregnancy. Omega-3 fatty acids prevent these processes from spinning out of control. Women deficient in omega-3 fatty acids, for instance, have, on average, shorter pregnancies, presumably because the overabundance of omega-6–derived prostaglandins promotes earlier labor and delivery.

Tipping the Balance

This elegant design, honed to perfection through eons of evolution, has gone awry. With the gradual phasing out of traditional foods and the advent of modern methods of food production in the past century, the Western diet has changed. Our bodies and minds evolved to use roughly equal parts omega-6 and omega-3 fatty acids, and the current overabundance of the omega-6 class has altered our internal physiology in ways we are just now beginning to understand. The good news is that this trend can most likely be reversed through dietary changes or supplements.

Populations maintaining historic omega-6 to omega-3 ratios (approximately 1 to 1) are protected from many of the scourges of the modern age. Greenland Eskimos eating their traditional diet of fish, whale, and seal, for example, have extremely low rates of heart disease. Their blood tests reveal a biochemical signature for cardiac health, including high levels of protective HDL cholesterol, low levels of LDL cholesterol, low levels of triglyceride, and low levels of platelet aggregation (stickiness), a risk factor for heart attack. Likewise, researchers have found that the fish-eating inhabitants of a typical Japanese fishing village had far lower rates of heart disease and arterial plaque than residents of a typical farming village who ate less fish.

Trends in major depression parallel those seen in cardiac disease. Another recently published study shows that in Japan, Hong Kong, and Taiwan, where fish consumption is high, rates of depression are extremely low—some ten times lower than in the United States. Even when one considers underreporting of psychiatric illnesses in some Asian cultures, major depression appears to be extremely rare in Japan, where omega-3 fatty acids in fish are consumed in great abundance.

Fat Brains, Healthy Minds

What happens to your brain when you change the balance of omega-6 to omega-3 from 1-to-1 to 20-to-1? Well, there are many ways a deficiency in omega-3s could affect mood, starting first with a change in the overall composition of the brain. In fact, the findings associating omega-3 consumption with depression and mood make sense in light of the brain's requirement for more omega-3 fatty acids than any other system in the body. Indeed, while the musculoskeletal system is rich in protein and minerals, the major structural component of the brain and its cells (other than water) is fat. The dry weight of an adult human brain is about 600 grams of lipid per kilogram, or an astounding 60 percent. Indeed, while other organ systems can function (if not optimally) on an omega-6 to omega-3 ratio of some 4 to 1, the brain may work best when fueled with equal quantities of the two essential fats.

The brain's needs are further complicated by its inability to use some forms of omega-3 fatty acids commonly found in the diet. Some organ systems can incorporate the shorter, eighteen-chain omega-3 precursor, called alpha-linolenic acid (ALA), found in green leafy vegetables, flaxseed, canola oil, and walnuts. But the human brain has an absolute requirement for the longer-chain omega-3 fatty acids: eicosapentanoic acid and docosahexa-noic acid, both found primarily in fish oil.

The studies have been somewhat mixed, but it appears that adult humans cannot convert enough ALA to EPA and then to DHA. Newborns appear to be better able to transform ALA to the longer-chain omega-3s, but these conversions may still be inadequate to fill the huge need of young children for omega-3 fatty acids. Thus, some nutritional scientists believe we must consume the fish and fish oil–derived long-chain omega-3s directly for optimal brain health. Strict vegetarians likely have lower levels of the long-chain omega-3 fatty acids, EPA and DHA, than nonvegetarians, but may in the future be able to purchase both EPA and DHA supplements derived directly from algae.

With sufficient quantities of EPA and DHA in the diet, the membranes surrounding our brain cells perform their crucial functions normally. In addition, the eicosanoids, the circulating hormones derived from omega-3 and omega-6 fatty acids, appear to have a vital, though still poorly understood, role in the brain, particularly in areas regulating mood. It is possible that high levels of EPA circulating in the blood or incorporated into membranes may be necessary for normal brain function, thus sustaining mood and possibly preventing or mitigating the symptoms of psychiatric disorders. Without sufficient quantities of EPA and DHA in the diet, brain cells use substitute lipids such as omega-6 and monounsaturated fatty acids, which have vastly different properties from the omega-3s.

Brain cells without sufficient quantities of omega-3 fatty acids in membranes have been shown to be dysfunctional in animal studies. Showing how and to what extent this deficiency compromises the health of the human brain will be an important goal for neuroscientists over the next few years.

The membrane is also an electrical regulator, controlling the movement of charged ions such as sodium and potassium into and out of the cell. Finally, the lipid bilayer serves as a doorway to the cell, controlling the movement of molecules and information in an organized fashion. Lipid bilayers composed of proper amounts of omega-3 fatty acids appear to function best.

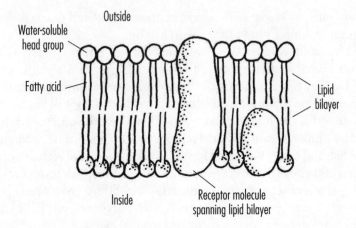

FIGURE 2–4: The Cell Membrane

The neuron, or brain cell, like all other cells, is enclosed by a membrane. The cell membrane is comprised of a double layer, or bilayer, of fats linked to other compounds that act as a highly selective barrier, preventing the contents of the cell from mixing with the rest of the body. The composition of the fats in the lipid bilayer have an enormous influence over the function of the cell. Neurons are intended to have very high levels of omega-3 fatty acids in their membranes.

Deficit of the Millennium

Why haven't we recognized the omega-3 deficiency? Historically, we have been slow to recognize nutritional deficiencies in the past. The story of vitamin C is particularly telling. Today we know that vitamin C deficiency in the diet leads to scurvy, an ancient, often-lethal condition marked by skin lesions, bloody vomiting, and death. But this was not clear to the nations of Western Europe when, from the 1400s on, they launched their sailing ships across the seas. Without adequate rations of fruits and vegetables, missions lost large numbers of crewmen to scurvy. No one knew the cause.

Finally, in 1747, an English naval surgeon named James Lind tested six remedies on sailors and discovered that oranges and lemons delivered a cure. His classic studies, published in 1753, are generally considered the first to prove that an essential food element can prevent a disease. Another fifty years would pass before the British Navy required rations of lemons or limes on sailing vessels. Scientists would not discover the vitamin C molecule (ascorbic acid) itself until 1932, when Charles Glenn King and W. A. Waugh of the University of Pittsburgh isolated the crystalline substance from lemon juice.

Unlike scurvy, the problems resulting from omega-3 fatty acid deficiency are more subtle and relatively new in human history, having emerged in force only in the past hundred years or so. The symptoms of omega-3 deficiency appear to be diverse and, in the case of the psychiatric disorders, so insidious that it may take medical science decades to pin them all down.

Studies tracing omega-3 fatty acid deficiency to increasing rates of heart disease are well established. Research linking omega-3 deficiency to depression and bipolar disorder, among other ills, is relatively new. The body of scientific literature describing this deficiency is large and varied, deriving from many sources and specialties. Although the literature, in aggregate, presents a powerful and compelling case of the hypothesis, most of the data are still indirect, and cause and effect have not been definitely established in many areas.

As researchers link deficits in these essential fatty acids to specific health problems, they will swiftly and accurately put appropriate treatments in place. Although our work is in its early stages, we have already begun the process in our patients with depression and manic depression and other psychiatric disorders, and as findings continue to come out, other medical specialties are now also exploring the power of the omega-3 essential fatty acids.

3

The Evolution Story

〜 When paleontologist Richard Leakey and his team discovered a two-million-year-old hominid skull, dubbed number 1470, on the eastern shore of Kenya's Lake Turkana, they helped settle one of science's most controversial issues: when and where the genus Homo had evolved. Leakey's dramatic find showed that one of our first human ancestors, Homo habilis, emerged at least two million years ago, around the enormous freshwater lakes in what is today known as the Rift Valley of East Africa.

Paleontologists now say that not one but at least three hominid species lived side by side around the shores of the East African lakes. Just one of those species was on the evolutionary line leading to a large-brained creature with higher intelligence: modern humans. In the quest to understand the forces driving human evolution, scientists continue to ask: What set that early human species apart from the two other hominid lines?

The latest theory is that human brain evolution was propelled forward not only by the development of opposable thumbs and the ability to walk on two legs but also by diet, which played a pivotal role. Analysis of dental fossils reveals that the three groups of hominids could coexist because they had vastly different diets. These diverse dietary requirements placed each hominid species in a unique ecological niche, reducing competition for food. A large-toothed species apparently maintained a coarse, fibrous, plant diet. A small-toothed species specialized in small fruits and berries as well as occasional rodents and eggs. But the third species—the one called Homo habilis, or "handy man," because of the primitive tool artifacts it left—was markedly omnivorous, consuming not just fruit and vegetables but also meat and fish.

Today, a quarter of a century after the discovery around the lakes of East Africa, the interest in Paleolithic nutrition has hit a new stride. The explosion of research is due in part to evidence that modern humans are very similar to the late hunter-gatherers who apparently evolved from Homo habilis to wander the earth in the Paleolithic era, some forty thousand years ago. Despite the fact that our ancestors evolved to function best on their Stone Age diet, in the last thousand years, and especially the last century, that diet has been radically changed. In the context of evolutionary time, one thousand years is a mere blip—enough for culture and menus to change, of course, but far too little for natural selection to introduce any significant change in our genes. Our biology probably cannot accommodate such an abrupt change without serious consequences.

The problem here is obvious: if the current diet differs from the diet we evolved to exploit, it may introduce unexpected and undesirable physiological changes. This altered physiology, researchers have begun to realize, could be responsible for many modern diseases, from atherosclerosis to depression to cancer. Could the Paleolithic diet be the true nutritional gold standard we should be following today? In sorting through such questions, scientists have discovered a dramatic discrepancy between modern and ancestral levels of the omega-3 fatty acids, an essential nutrient in the diet. There is substantial evidence to support the notion that omega-3 fatty acids, so abundant in the Stone Age, were essential to the evolution of the brain.

It is impossible to go back in time literally, of course, but researchers wielding a host of scientific tools have gone back indirectly, assembling some probable Stone Age dietary patterns along the way. One technique focuses on modern hunter-gatherer populations with diets closer to that of our evolutionary past. It was the classic study of Greenland Eskimos, conducted in the 1970s that drew attention to high concentrations of omega-3 fatty acids in their diets, ultimately linking the omega-3s to low rates of heart disease. In a more recent study of Yupik Eskimos living in southwestern Alaska, scientists found an advantage to a diet high in salmon, marine mammals, and other sources of omega-3 fatty acids. These Eskimos succumbed to circulatory disease at only one-third the rate of those on modern Western diets in the United States. However, an important caveat is that these studies did not look at other factors, such as exercise levels, which are known to have an impact on heart disease.

The Eskimo diet is extremely limited due to a lack of food diversity (particularly plants) in the harsh arctic environment, especially compared to the one around the East African lakes. However, another group of modern hunter-gatherers—the Australian Aborigines—consumes a more varied fare, from various vegetables and seeds to wild animals and fish. The Aborigines are of special interest to nutritionists because they show little or no evidence of diabetes and cardiovascular disease in their natural environment, yet suffer as much as the rest of us when adopting the diet and lifestyle of the West. Looking into the phenomenon, nutrition researchers Joan M. Naughton and Kerin O'Dea of the Royal Melbourne Hospital and Andrew J. Sinclair of the Royal Melbourne Institute of Technology traced the Aboriginal advantage to traditional foods, especially the levels and types of fat in their diet.

The scientists analyzed the traditional Aboriginal diet across a wide range of geographic regions, from the tropical coast of the north through the vast, arid center to the cooler climates of the south. The specific foods varied greatly, with some Aborigines getting as much as 64 percent of their calories from animal foods. But even in this last group, saturated fat in the diet is uniformly low and the essential fatty acid content, including omega-3 and omega-6 fatty acids, fairly high. This is because wild game have very little saturated fat and relatively high levels of essential fatty acids when compared to domesticated animals. This fatty acid profile is a consequence of the wild animal species' consumption of wild plants containing high levels of polyunsaturated fatty acids. This is analogous to the absence of omega-3 fatty acids in farm-raised fish versus wild fish if the "domesticated" fish are not fed nutrients from the sea.

Out of the Wild

What is true for Aborigines may be extended to preagricultural hunter-gatherer populations across the world. Whether the source of meat is Pacific black duck, red-bellied black snake, bluebone fish, or crocodile, wild animals, unlike their domesticated counterparts, are lean and contain higher amounts of omega-3. The farm-bred livestock of today are reared in confined conditions on a high-carbohydrate grain diet enriched with saturated fat, which may be one of the reasons that the meat we consume from them is high in this unhealthy lipid as well. But wild animals, free to roam and eat what they want without human interference, do not develop the same fatty deposits. Instead, much of the fat they contain is structural—the polyunsaturated kind used to build cell membranes and muscles, a mix of the essential fatty acids, omega-6 and omega-3. As we may come to see, the type of fat itself can influence whether the body gains weight—as with saturated fat—or burns more energy as heat—as is the case with the omega-3 fatty acids.

Fat Infiltration: Wild Game Versus Commercial Meat

Deposits of highly saturated fat have infiltrated animal food sources over the years as some species have become increasingly domesticated. In contrast, essential fatty acids, including a balance of omega-6 and omega-3, increase dramatically when animals live freely in the wild. Fat in wild game contains roughly three times as many polyunsaturated fatty acids as fat in commercial meat, reflecting the increased storage fat that accumulates in domestic meat animals. In addition, wild game has seven times more omega-3 fatty acids than commercial meat.

To reach these conclusions, Michael A. Crawford of the University of North London studied a range of species, including the giraffe. He found that for giraffes reared in a zoo, the fat profile matched that of other domesticated animals reared in captivity. This was in stark contrast to two giraffes of similar age roaming the wild area of Nabiswa, Sebei, in Uganda. "The zoo giraffes were traditionally fed on hay and some concentrated nutrients while the wild giraffes had access to a variety of trees," Crawford explained. The kernel of fruit from one of those tree species, Balanites aegyptiaca, was 20 percent oil by weight, and more than 50 percent of the oil was of the polyunsaturated essential fatty acid class.

Yet other research shows that frequently consumed vegetables of eras past were loaded with omega-3 fatty acids too. One such vegetable source now out of favor is the spinachlike purslane, recently studied by Artemis P. Simopoulos, M.D., and her colleagues at the Center for Genetics, Nutrition, and Health in Washington, D.C. The Simopoulos team found purslane to be the richest source of the shorter-chain omega-3 fatty acid ALA of any green leafy vegetable yet examined. Her group even detected small quantities of the omega-3 fatty acids EPA and DHA thought to be present only in food from fresh and salt water. Hardly a common item on the modern grocery list, purslane grows in the wild, where it has become one of the most frequently reported weeds in the world.

If purslane is considered an annoying weed today, our ancestors had a different point of view. Present in Europe since prehistoric times, purslane was naturally harvested from the wild as food. Recognized not just for its nutritional value but also for its healing powers, Hippocratic physicians used it to treat headaches, stomach and intestinal ills, heart problems, inflammatory problems, and shortness of breath. In addition to purslane, other long-forgotten wild plant foods, including hoary cress, goosefoot, and plantain, are rich sources of omega-3 oils as well.

Produced by cells of land- and water-based plants, essential polyunsaturated fatty acids were plentiful during the Paleolithic era that ushered in the ascent of modern humans. This widespread availability may explain why humans (along with other animals) either never evolved or lost through evolution the enzymes needed to synthesize these essential fatty acids themselves. In the evolutionary crucible of the Paleolithic period, between ten thousand and forty thousand years ago, the abundance of omega-3 fatty acids, in particular, appears to have been essential in sculpting Homo sapiens as we appear today. Both omega-3 and omega-6 fatty acids were bountiful in the wild, leafy plants consumed by roaming animals; and the long-chain omega-3s, EPA and DHA, so essential to the function of the brain, were manufactured by algae (also known as phytoplankton), the single-celled plants floating in freshwater lakes and living in the seas. Zooplankton, tiny single-celled animal organisms, ate the phytoplankton. In turn, shrimplike organisms called krill ate the zooplankton, and small fish and whales ate the krill. Omega-3 fatty acids traveled through this and other food chains, eventually reaching Stone Age humans (see Figure 3–1).

To the Stone Age and Back

The diet of the Stone Age is highly relevant because it is the diet we were born to consume. Our genetic composition suggests that the diet we consumed in ancient times—the diet we evolved to use—might still be best. For nearly all of human existence, evolutionary forces maintained an appropriate relationship between our ancestors' physiological requirements and their diet, according to Emory University anthropologist and radiologist S. Boyd Eaton, M.D. But starting in the agricultural revolution of ten thousand years ago and accelerating through the Industrial Revolution of the late eighteenth century, genetic evolution

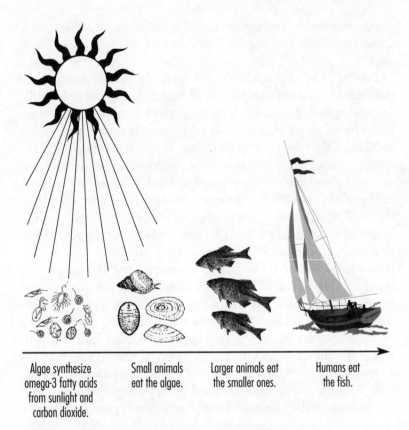

Algae synthesize
omega-3 fatty acids
from sunlight and
carbon dioxide.

Small animals
eat the algae.

Larger animals eat
the smaller ones.

Humans eat
the fish.

FIGURE 3–1: Omega-3 Fatty Acids and the Food Chain

The omega-3 fatty acids are made only in plants. Vertebrate animals either never evolved the ability to synthesize omega-3s or lost that ability somewhere along the evolutionary path. The largest source of omega-3 fatty acids in the ocean and freshwater bodies of water are algae, single-celled plants that use the energy from sunlight to convert carbon dioxide and water into complex biochemicals, including the omega-3 fatty acids. Small aquatic animals, such as shrimp, feed on the algae, assimilating the omega-3 fatty acids into their bodies. Larger, predatory fish feed on the shrimp and the process continues through various food chains all the way to humans.

has been unable to keep pace with changes in human living conditions, including our altered nutritional patterns.

Changes in our society as a result of the agricultural and Industrial revolutions included huge population growth and a shift from the farm to the city for many people. These changes, as well as rapid advances in food production technology, have led to the dramatic shift away from our ancestral diets. Addressing this issue recently, Dr. Alexander Leaf, a cardiologist at Massachusetts General Hospital, reiterated the famous eighteenth-century biologist Malthus's proposition that food has always been a limiting factor in population growth. Leaf notes that humans were not always as successful in conquering the earth's resources as we are today. It took until 1850 for the human population to reach one billion and another 150 years to grow to the six billion it is today. It is through revolutionary new techniques for food production—irrigation, fertilizers, farm machinery, pesticides, and, most recently, genetic modification—as well as politics and economics, that we have the ability to keep the multitudes fed.

But while quantity increased, it has only recently become apparent that the quality of our diet has declined. Most nutritionists and physicians today agree that the diet adopted by Western societies over the past hundred years has contributed to the drastic increase in the risk of coronary heart disease, hypertension, obesity, diabetes, and some types of cancer. "These conditions have emerged as dominant health problems only in the last century," says Leaf, "and are virtually unknown among the few surviving hunter-gatherer populations whose way of life and eating habits most closely resemble those of preagricultural human beings." Leaf does not believe we can attribute the rates of these illnesses to the longer average life span today. "The members of technologically primitive cultures who survive to the age of sixty years or more," he says, "remain relatively free of these disorders, unlike their *civilized* counterparts."

One could also wonder whether the profound reduction in physical activity since the Industrial Revolution has contributed to our species' health problems. Our Stone Age ancestors certainly had, on average, hours more "exercise" than we have today. If one adds high levels of omega-3 fatty acids to the Ornish diet (see Chapter 2), it may be the closest thing to our biologically ideal diet.

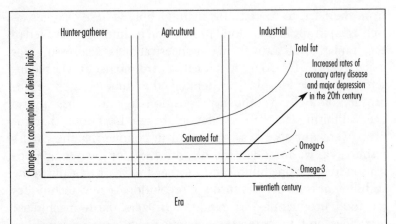

FIGURE 3–2: Dietary Lipid Changes Through the Ages

This graph illustrates the changes in dietary fats that might have occurred during human history. The speculative data for the prehistorical portion of the graph were derived from modern hunter-gatherer populations whose diets may resemble those of our Paleolithic-era ancestors. Note the increased consumption of total fat, saturated fat, and omega-6 fatty acids, with a corresponding decline in dietary omega-3 fatty acids during the twentieth century. Accompanying these dietary lipid changes, coronary artery disease (CAD) has increased dramatically during the past one hundred years. There are many possible reasons for the rise in heart disease, but the loss of omega-3 fatty acids and the other changes in dietary lipids may be a major factor. As will be discussed later in the book, the progressive increase in the prevalence of major depression in the twentieth century closely parallels the rise in CAD. This finding suggests a role for dietary lipid changes, particularly omega-3 depletion, in the changing rates of major depression.

S. Boyd Eaton estimates that in the late Paleolithic period, our ancestors consumed 3,000 calories a day—35 percent meat and 65 percent vegetable. Despite the high intake of animal protein, fat intake was relatively low (wild game is very lean), with high proportions of polyunsaturated fatty acid, including plenty of omega-3 fatty acids. Today, similar quantities of omega-3 fatty acids are consumed by only a few groups, including Eskimos and inhabitants of Japanese fishing villages (see Table 3–1).

TABLE 3-1: Comparison of a Paleolithic Diet to Modern Diets

This table represents a rough comparison of several modern diets with the diet believed to represent what our evolutionary ancestors ate, based on dental fossils, the diets of modern hunter-gatherer populations, and other indirect evidence. Note how the traditional diets of the Japanese, the Australian Aborigines, and the native peoples in the Arctic regions of North America are similar in omega-3 content to the postulated Paleolithic diet. In contrast, note how the modern Western diet is virtually devoid of omega-3 fatty acids.

In the table, the number zero represents none while the plus signs represent progressively increasing quantities, with + meaning minimal and ++++ meaning large amounts.

FOOD	OMEGA-3 FATTY ACID CONTENT	PALEOLITHIC HUMAN DIET	MODERN U.S. DIET	MODERN JAPANESE DIET	TRADITIONAL INUIT DIET	TRADITIONAL AUSTRALIAN ABORIGINAL DIET
Domesticated animals	0	0	+++	+	0	0
Dairy products	0	+/-	+++	+	0	+/-
Processed foods	0	0	+++	++	0	0
Cultivated grains	0	0	+++	++	0	0
Cultivated greens	+/-	0	++	++	0	0
Wild game	++	++	+/-	0	++	++
Wild greens	+	+++	0	0	+	++
Fish	++++	++	+	+++	+++	++

"Our experience in the Paleolithic has continuing relevance," says Eaton, because the period from 35,000 to 15,000 years ago may be "the last time the human gene pool functioned within the nutritional parameters for which it had been originally selected." Michael Crawford, the nutritional scientist who compared the diets of wild game with domestic species, raised the red flag regarding the long-term destructive power of what he called "fat infiltration" and "artificial drift" as far back as the 1960s, before the idea of polyunsaturated fatty acids as essential foods had even taken hold. "It might be argued that animals have wide tolerance to changes in diet," said Crawford, but for humans, that "wide change has already occurred." Can the artificial drift from our original, balanced diet be justified, he asked, especially given the importance of essential fatty acids throughout the body and brain—in the structure of cell membranes, the production of prostaglandins and other signaling molecules, and a multitude of other biological functions? And does exceeding our limits of nutritional tolerance throw the body off-balance, invoking unexpected types of disease? In short, if the diet of the Paleolithic was evolutionary, could today's diet be *devolutionary*—possibly reversing the progression of mankind?

How to Feed an Evolving Brain

Such questions are especially relevant in light of new research into the evolution of the human brain, which tripled in size over the past three million years. Seeking to explain the brain's explosive growth, paleoanthropologists have proposed the existence of a number of reciprocal evolutionary forces, all acting together to propel the emergence of modern humans: the upright, bipedal stance, enabling negotiation of complex environments and freeing the forelimbs for other tasks; the hand with an opposable thumb, enabling tool building and tool use; and the development of speech and increased intelligence, facilitating communication. There is no question that these developments were crucial to the processes driving our evolution, but recently emerging research suggests that diet itself was the gatekeeper—the one element that could permit an increase in brain size or derail the process.

A larger, more intelligent brain can occur only under optimal conditions. The reason is that larger brains come at a cost. A large brain relative to body size requires more energy to develop and sustain it over the life of the organism. In addition, large amounts of omega-3 and omega-6 long-chain essential fatty acids are needed for optimal structure of the brain. Researchers comparing relative brain size to metabolic rate have found that humans expend about three or four times more energy sustaining their brain than other primate species. Small-brained species can spend the entire day foraging for low-quality foods like leaves in trees, but big-brained species spend time doing other things: building tools and societies, creating art, teaching and rearing our young. To enable these higher aspirations, our ancestors had to develop better and more efficient means of feeding their expanding brain. The one way to come by the extra energy in a limited time frame was to discover methods to obtain higher quality, calorically dense food—fare that provides more bang for the buck and saves time, too. Thus may have emerged a reciprocal and progressive process in which better quality food permitted a larger brain and the larger brain discovered even better ways to obtain even higher quality food.

This process might have become possible for early humans about 2.5 million years ago, when a vast, global cooling dramatically increased the amount of open grassland in Africa, reducing the density and changing the distribution of plant foods, thus making animals, including fish, an increasingly attractive food resource. Some of the hominid species maintained diets high in fruit resources, but our direct ancestors increasingly relied on fish, opening the doorway for rapid evolution of the brain. If we required even higher octane nutrition to step up from early Homo to Homo sapiens, as evolutionary biologists have recently suggested, there is one place where we could have met those requirements: Africa's Rift Valley, with its enormous freshwater lakes.

Altered long ago by the only volcano known to have erupted carbonatite (a form of carbonate rock, comprised of carbon and oxygen), these carbon-rich proto-seas gave rise to unique populations of freshwater fish and shellfish, species with essential fatty acid ratios more like that of the human brain than any other food source known. Although protein, vitamins, and trace elements were also important for brain development, it is becoming accepted that the increased availability of long-chain essential fatty acids, especially DHA and EPA, were the nutritional drivers of explosive brain growth. Without abundant sources of long-chain omega-3 fatty acids, the uniquely complex human nervous system could not have developed, no matter what other factors had come into play. The abundance of omega-3 fatty acid food sources may have made the Rift Valley an ideal setting for rapid evolution of the human brain.

The latest elaboration of this theory has emerged from the international team of C. Leigh Broadhurst of the Human Nutrition Center at the U.S. Department of Agriculture, Stephen C. Cunnane of the University of Toronto, and London's Michael Crawford. They start with the evolutionist's proverbial question: Which came first, the chicken or the egg? "Did hominids 'become' intelligent enough to begin fishing," the researchers ask, "or did they fish and then become intelligent?" These two possibilities need not be mutually exclusive, Broadhurst concludes. Instead, since the two options reinforce each other, the answer lies in a reciprocal push-pull that hominids scavenged and caught fish opportunistically, a process that helped increase intelligence enough for them to fish more often and more successfully. For instance, a common Rift Valley phenomenon known as fish stranding—in which fish become trapped in shallow pools of water—enabled hominids to club or spear them, and that ability, combined with bipedality, opposable thumbs, language, and other factors, resulted in larger brains and greater intelligence, enabling, among other activities, more aggressive forms of fishing and still more omega-3 oils in the diet.

Human Family Tree

Some 3.8 to 3.9 million years ago, an early human ancestor, *Australopithecus afarensis*, the oldest widespread hominid, roamed the East African Rift Valley. Most paleontologists now believe that between 2.3 and 2.5 million years ago, *A. afarensis*, or some other common ancestor, gave rise to three species: *Australopithecus boisei*, *Australopithecus robustus*, and some form of *Homo*, most likely *Homo habilis*. About 1.5 million years ago, *H. habilis* in turn gave rise to a number of species, including *Homo erectus* and *Homo heidelbergensis*. Until fairly recently, paleontologists thought that *H. erectus* gave rise to *Homo neanderthalensis* (Neanderthal man) and *Homo sapiens*. But the latest evidence indicates *H. erectus* was an evolutionary dead end while *H. heidelbergensis* was the common ancestor to Neanderthals and modern humans.

It is notable that while fossils of all these species have been found in numerous areas of the East African Rift Valley, *A. boisei* and *A. robustus* lived in enclosed forest areas as well as along the lake margins. *Homo*, on the other hand, has been found almost exclusively around the margins of the lakes. As time went on, dental fossils reveal, *A. boisei* and *A. robustus* became increasingly adaptive to arboreal niches and diets while *H. habilis* ultimately evolved into *Homo sapiens*.

Evidence linking the rise of *Homo sapiens* to a diet rich in fish and other aquatic food sources is clear in the fossil record of the Rift Valley. Modern human fossils dating to about a hundred thousand years ago are surrounded by the shells of mussels, turbans, and periwinkles. Some of the shells are burned, indicating that the fish was cooked. Those eating habits continued for tens of thousands of years, with evidence of progressive technological development. More recent fossils of *Homo sapiens* inhabiting the

East African Rift Valley forty thousand years ago, for instance, have been found with barbed spear points and evidence for fish-trapping dams and weirs. There is evidence that foraging groups returned to certain areas year after year, perhaps to take advantage of spawning runs or seasonal fish strandings.

"Since sophisticated fishing tackle, harpoons, and fishhooks are usually not found up to eighteen thousand years ago," says Broadhurst, "it has been assumed that earlier humans and hominids did not eat fish. While they may not have actively fished, they may well have eaten fish." Fish scavenging and shellfish gathering is not possible in every environment, "but it is very plausible in the unique East African Rift Valley, and in other areas of Africa with long histories of hominid occupation."

There is no question that our ancestors evolved from tool users to tool makers to fine craftsmen and organized societies with astonishing rapidity, paralleling a dramatic increase in brain size from the early days of *Homo habilis* to the emergence of *Homo sapiens*. It is difficult to explain this in an evolutionary sense, says Broadhurst, without at least considering the brain-specific nutrients available to early *Homo*. "Grabbing or trapping fish and crustaceans by hand and smashing mollusk shells requires less sophistication than either hunting or scavenging game, yet yields a far greater amount of the preformed docosahexanoic acid (DHA, omega-3) and arachidonic acid (AA, omega-6) for the effort."

In the end, says the Broadhurst team, it is impossible to explain the human cerebral cortex without an ancient abundance of preformed long-chain fatty acids, especially the omega-3s. Of course, the human species expanded beyond the fertile lake cradle that propelled its growth. But we could not have left without the ability to adapt to diverse environments and extract from those areas other sources of omega-3 fatty acids.

The Future of Evolution

If omega-3 fatty acids were so pivotal to the emergence of the human brain, what will happen as we systematically remove them from the nutritional mix? Increasingly credible research suggests that lack of abundant and balanced essential fatty acids in utero can lead to lowered IQ scores and diminished visual skills. Emerging research has now postulated that omega-3 fatty acid deficiency leads to an increased risk for depression, bipolar disorder, attention deficit–hyperactivity disorder (ADHD), and possibly violence. Physical consequences of omega-3 fatty acid deficiency, including heart disease and rheumatoid arthritis, are now well documented. As severe as these problems may seem today, they may get worse if we do not address them now.

Some experts think that by controlling our environment, we have halted our own evolution. By modifying the world to fit ourselves, we have interfered with the process of natural selection, in which individuals most suited to the unyielding requirements of nature are more likely to survive and reproduce. These experts say human evolution is now metabiological, or in the realm of ideas; in other words, instead of evolving in sync with the natural world, we change through interaction with technology, culture, and other products of the mind.

But new insights into the Stone Age diet show this leap to a new evolutionary paradigm may have to wait. For while we have modified the world to fit an image of ourselves, we have apparently lacked the wisdom to do it right. The dietary milieu we have created may be deficient in the single nutrient possibly responsible for our prodigious brains.

What does this mean for us? If we are biologically identical to our Paleolithic ancestors, then we cannot expect today's processed food to propel the human brain and intellect in the right direction or even sustain them for long. In an interesting discovery, scientists have found evidence that our dramatic increase in brain size has not just slowed but possibly reversed; indeed, the human brain is some 10 percent smaller than it was just a century ago, though the significance of this is unclear. This apparent shrinkage may be linked to many factors, including possibly the widespread shortage of omega-3 fatty acids experienced over recent generations. Other studies described later in this book show increased rates of depression at increasingly younger ages of onset with each passing decade of the twentieth century.

We have sought to explain this trend in terms of social systems, but we could, in addition, look more carefully at the nutrients in our foods affecting our brains and mood.

As instructive as the Stone Age diet is, we cannot incorporate it wholesale into the lives we live today. Our Paleolithic ancestors required about 75 percent more calories than we do for all that hunting, scavenging, and gathering; and even at those levels, the burn rate was so high that their body fat measurements were probably outrageously low by today's standards. What is more, the freshwater fish and shellfish of the African cradle were not contaminated with mercury or synthetic carcinogenic chemicals, an unpleasant artifact of our technological age. Today, eating one can of tuna per week would not provide enough long-chain omega-3 fatty acids, and more than this may be hazardous to human health.

For humans to succeed in the twenty-first century, several factors must be present: a continued explosion of high technology, a favorable political and economic climate, population control, a reduction in environmental pollution, and quite possibly a return to our ancient dietary roots, most notably including larger quantities of omega-3 fatty acids.

4

The Wellness Molecules: Omega-3 Fatty Acids and Health

୶ We have come to accept illness and infirmity as the natural order of aging. As we grow older, we might succumb to heart disease, stroke, or cancer. If we escape these killers into old age, such scourges as Alzheimer's disease, arthritis, diabetes, and obesity may compromise the quality of life, if not the quantity of days.

In the late 1970s, a medical establishment convinced of this legacy was amazed to find that modern hunter-gatherer groups like the Inuit lived relatively free of such problems—but only if they maintained traditional diet and exercise regimes, avoiding the foods and lifestyle of the West. The Inuit advantage was attributed to the very long-chain omega-3 fatty acids, EPA and DHA, found in their food staples of fatty fish and fish-eating marine mammals like whales and seals.

Since these surprising findings were documented, researchers have reported a healing role for omega-3 fatty acids across a broad spectrum of disorders and disease. They have been shown to reduce the risk of coronary artery disease and cardiac sudden death; mitigate the pain and disability of Crohn's disease; lower blood pressure; diminish the pain and stiffness in rheumatoid arthritis; reduce triglycerides; counteract or prevent symptoms of asthma; improve the health of insulin-dependent diabetics; and possibly perform many other clinical actions. In fact, the omega-3s may prevent or delay the onset of these modern diseases.

Omega-3 fatty acids have so many biological roles because they are a primary element of health for virtually every cell and organ system in the body. Along with their partners, the omega-6 fatty acids, they keep our bodies in balance, modulating such basic physiological functions as inflammation, cell signaling, blood pressure, immune response, the electrical excitability of heart and brain cells, and cell death.

This chapter examines how decades of research across numerous medical specialties and scientific disciplines has begun to clarify the role of omega-3 fatty acids in many of the most troubling health problems today. Only now are we beginning to understand the profound importance and complexity of the omega-3 and omega-6 system throughout the body.

Omega-3 Oils and the Healthy Heart

There are any number of potentially fatal diseases, from lupus to cancer, but the number-one killer in Western industrialized countries is heart disease. Despite significant improvements in treatment since the 1960s, heart disease kills about half a million Americans each year (compare this to the 57,000 U.S. military deaths during the Vietnam War), and half of the sudden cardiac deaths occur in people with no previously known heart disease.

By now, most people know that a diet high in saturated fat and cholesterol increases the risk for heart disease, but the newest evidence shows that not all fat is bad. However, the early focus by the American Heart Association on saturated fat and cholesterol as causing heart disease ignored other factors, such as the inflammatory aspects of coronary artery disease driven by omega-6 fatty acids unchecked by omega-3s. Without an abundance of omega-3s, the omega-6 arachidonic acid promotes atherosclerosis, heart attack, and fatal cardiac arrythmias. Also unrecognized were the numerous additional lifesaving benefits of the omega-3 fatty acids themselves. When it comes to the heart, diets high in omega-3 fatty acids appear to be the healthiest of all.

A Closer Look

Heart attacks (myocardial infarction) occur when coronary arteries supplying oxygen-laden blood to the heart muscle itself become blocked due to atherosclerosis, sudden constriction of the coronary arteries, blood clots, or other causes. When one or more coronary arteries are blocked, oxygen cannot reach the region of the heart supplied by the blocked artery. If the lack of oxygen (known as ischemia) continues for more than a few minutes, the affected heart cells die. The specific heart region affected and the extent of the tissue damage determine the severity of the myocardial infarction and whether it will be fatal. Even if the ischemic damage to the heart muscle is not severe, the electrical signaling system that coordinates the effective pumping action of the heart may turn chaotic, leading to a fatal arrhythmia, often referred to as cardiac sudden death. Omega-3s reduce the rate of fatal arrhythmias by 30 percent. In the United States alone, more than 70,000 lives could be saved each year if Americans had sufficient omega-3s in their bodies.

The underlying cause of most heart disease is atherosclerosis. Inflammation caused by the omega-6 fatty acid counterpart of EPA, known as arachidonic acid, is a major factor initiating the development of atherosclerotic plaques inside the coronary arteries. Plaques are abnormal deposits of cholesterol and other biochemicals that can build up on the inside of a coronary artery damaged by inflammation, eventually forming a fibrous, fatty thickening and leading to atherosclerosis, also known as "hardening of the arteries." Ultimately, the plaque will produce a narrowing or a complete blockage of the coronary artery, leading to myocardial infarction. Another complication of excessive levels of omega-6 fatty acids is that arachidonic acid tends to increase the aggregation of platelets, which causes blood clots to form (thrombosis). If the thrombus is large enough, blood flow will be blocked, leading to myocardial infarction. Conversely, EPA reduces platelet stickiness and clotting.

EPA and DHA also prevent or conceivably could reverse plaque buildup by raising levels of HDL (high-density lipoprotein, or "good" cholesterol). HDL transports cholesterol away from the arteries back to the liver, where it can be degraded. EPA also lowers triglycerides, which are now being recognized as an additional risk factor for the development of cardiovascular disease.

The omega-3 fatty acids and their eicosanoid derivatives are further known for their ability to relax and dilate blood vessels (including the coronary arteries), thus increasing blood flow. This vasodilation may additionally protect against myocardial infarction by increasing blood flow to the heart.

EPA and the Platelet Aggregation

The heart-protecting ability of EPA to reduce the stickiness of platelets and decrease the formation of blood clots is one of EPA's most important health benefits. However, this ability to reduce the formation of potentially fatal clots within blood vessels has often been misunderstood and has raised concerns that omega-3 fatty acids could cause bleeding to occur in the body. This concern presumably arises because aspirin, which also decreases platelet aggregation and blood clotting, is known to cause occasional abnormal bleeding. In fact, no cases of bleeding from EPA or omega-3s have ever been documented. Supporting the safety of the omega-3 fatty acids is a study where participants receiving a high dosage of omega-3 fatty acids underwent either angioplasty or unsuccessful angioplasty followed by coronary artery bypass surgery. These cardiac procedures and surgery may cause substantial blood loss, yet the patients receiving omega-3 fatty acids suffered no excessive bleeding.

Understanding the difference between aspirin and EPA at the level of the platelet illustrates the beauty of nature's balance of the omega-3 and omega-6 fatty acids and why EPA is unlikely to lead to abnormal bleeding. Aspirin causes a nearly complete and permanent block of the platelets' ability to aggregate and form clots. The action of aspirin lasts for the life of the platelet, and because it is so complete, aspirin can cause abnormal bleeding. This is why aspirin should not be taken before surgery or in pregnancy unless specifically prescribed. EPA on the other hand, causes only a partial and time-limited reduction in platelet's ability to form clots. Recent research has shown that even a 17 gram dose of EPA (omega-3) produces a reversible inhibition of platelet aggregation of between 40 and 60 percent. Compare this partial action of a huge dose of EPA to the 99.9 percent irreversible inhibition of platelet function by a quarter tablet of aspirin. Aspirin causes an all-or-none action, which can cause problems in susceptible people. In contrast, EPA and its eicosanoid derivatives promote a state of health by preserving the normal ability of the body to stop bleeding, while competing with and limiting the ability of the arachidonic acid (omega-6–derived eicosanoids) to cause abnormal clotting within blood vessels. This system of checks and balances between EPA and arachidonic acid shows why it is so important to have as close to the one-to-one ratio of omega-6 and omega-3 that nature intended.

Preventing Heart Attacks: Omega-3s and the Mediterranean Diet

For years, the low-fat and "heart-healthy" diet of the American Heart Association recommended increasing the amount of vegetable and seed oils in the U.S. diet and reducing saturated fats and cholesterol. Reducing saturated fats and cholesterol has undoubtedly saved lives. But although vegetable and seed oils contain high quantities of omega-6 fatty acids, they have virtually no omega-3s. The effect has been to accelerate the imbalance of the omega-3 and omega-6 fatty acids. The widespread incorporation of omega-6–containing oils into the U.S. food supply has likely *increased* the risk of heart disease. Thus, the American Heart Association position seems to be in conflict with recent recommendations for the Mediterranean diet, which is high in monounsaturated and polyunsaturated (both omega-3 and omega-6) fats. Advocates for each strategy have cited different studies and statistics to bolster their views. In the end, the bottom line is this: if the high fat of the Mediterranean diet is *really* so healthy, the question is why.

No one questioned that Greeks, Italians, and other Southern Europeans on a traditional Mediterranean diet are at far lower risk for heart disease, cancer, and other health problems of other Western nations. But the interpretation of this finding was complex, especially in light of the multifaceted nature of the Mediterranean menu and other possible factors contributing to the low rates of these ills. Is the heart protected by plentiful fruits and vegetables and by monounsaturated fats like olive oil, or by something else entirely? In France, for instance, consumption of saturated fat is outrageously high, yet heart disease remains low. Experts call this situation the "French paradox," and some have suggested that some component of red wine, prominent in the French diet, plays a role. By the 1980s, most of the medical profession understood that coronary heart disease and nutrition are tightly linked, but cause and effect of different foods was difficult to determine. Without a clinical trial comparing a test group to controls, it was impossible to quantify the benefits of a particular diet or to pinpoint whether a specific nutrient protected the heart.

Not until 1994 did researchers in southern France provide more insight into the Mediterranean diet, and in the process they revealed that much of the benefit derived *not* from olive oil, as had been thought, but from omega-3 fatty acids. Among other questions, the study sought to determine why patients with heart disease seemed to accrue little benefit from olive oil, despite all the epidemiological evidence suggesting they should.

Spearheaded by Michel de Lorgeril and Serge Renaud of the Institut National de la Santé et de la Recherche Medicale (IN-SERM), the seminal Lyon Diet Heart Study focused on 605 patients who had survived their first heart attack. All the participants received state-of-the-art medical care from their physicians. They also received dietary advice.

The control group was placed on a presumably heart-healthy diet similar to that recommended by the American Heart Association. The experimental group was placed on a Mediterranean diet: more bread, more root and green vegetables, more fish, less meat, and plenty of fruit. Butter and cream were replaced not with olive oil, as in the control group, but with a canola-based margarine. This INSERM margarine was similar in composition to olive oil except it had more omega-3 fatty acids. The IN-SERM margarine was composed of 16.4 percent of the omega-6 oil, linoleic acid, versus 8.6 percent for olive oil, and 4.8 percent of the omega-3 oil alpha-linolenic acid, compared to only 0.6 percent for olive oil. Notably, the INSERM margarine had an omega-6 to omega-3 ratio of about 4 to 1. The addition of fish also raised the omega-3 content of the diet, lowering the omega-6 to omega-3 ratio still further. (The typical American diet has an overall omega-6 to omega-3 ratio of approximately 20 to 1.)

The findings, published in the prestigious medical journal *Lancet* in 1994, were striking. There were twenty deaths, including eight sudden deaths, in the thirty-three-member control group. For the thirty-eight participants on the special INSERM diet and margarine, by contrast, there were just eight deaths and not a single sudden death. The experimental group did so much better than the controls, says de Lorgeril, that ethics required stopping the study after just a year so that the control group could have access to the lifesaving strategy as well.

That is not the end of it. In a follow-up to the study, the researchers set out to determine whether those in the experimental group continued to comply with the diet and what benefits they received. Most had maintained the high omega-3 INSERM diet over the years, the study revealed, with 1.2 percent of them experiencing a cardiac event each year. In a separate control group of heart patients, by contrast, 4.1 percent experienced cardiac events in an identical time frame, an increase in cardiac incidents of more than 300 percent.

These extraordinary results are backed up by a series of studies examining exactly how omega-3 fatty acids affect the heart. The research reveals a powerful, multifaceted role. Indeed, while the low-fat diet of the American Heart Association works simply by lowering saturated fat and, by extension, the bad cholesterol (LDL), omega-3 oils do that and much more.

The definitive study of omega-3 fatty acids and heart disease was published in 1999 in the *Lancet*. Led by Roberto Marchioli, M.D. of GISSI-Prevenzione Coordinating Centre in Santa Maria Imbaro, Italy, the team studied 11,324 recent heart attack survivors from October 1993 to September 1995. Study participants were randomly assigned to one of four groups, where they received omega-3 fatty acids, vitamin E, both vitamin E and omega-3 fatty acids, or nothing. Each participant was followed for three and a half years. For these patients, already following a Mediterranean-style diet, the GISSI team found that vitamin E did not affect the outcome. But overwhelmingly, the researchers found, omega-3 fatty acids lowered risk for fatal as well as nonfatal heart attacks and stroke. Impressively, omega-3 fatty acid supplements decreased the risk of death from myocardial infarction some 30 percent. This study replicated the results of previous well-designed studies, firmly establishing the lifesaving qualities of the omega-3 fatty acids from fish oil.

Omega-3s Save Lives

- Reduced risk of first heart attack by 20 to 40 percent
- Reduced risk of sudden death during and after a heart attack by 20 to 40 percent
- Slightly lower blood pressure
- Reduction in serum triglycerides
- Reduction in LDL ("bad") cholesterol

Experts have highlighted other omega-3 fatty acid–associated benefits:

- *Lower blood pressure.* Study after study shows that omega-3 fatty acids help modestly to lower blood pressure, a major cause of heart disease. Omega-3 and omega-6 fatty acids are both converted to a group of substances known as eicosanoids. The body converts omega-6 fatty acids to the hormonelike eicosanoid thromboxane A2, a powerful constrictor of blood vessels, which raises blood pressure. Conversely, the omega-3s are converted to thromboxane A3, a vasodilator that competes with and reduces the impact of A2.

  Omega-3 fatty acids and omega-6 fatty acids directly compete for the same enzyme, which converts them into the thromboxanes. Thus, high levels of omega-6 fatty acids would lead to high levels of thromboxane A2, resulting in the constriction of arterioles (small arteries) and high blood pressure. By contrast, high levels of omega-3 fatty acids would lead to high levels of thromboxane A3, resulting in more relaxed arterioles and lower blood pressure. Blood vessels suddenly constricted due to thromboxane A2 are especially dangerous for those with the already narrowed blood vessels of atherosclerosis, greatly increasing risk for heart attack or stroke.

- Reduced risk of cardiac sudden death. In the aftermath of a heart attack, most of those who succumb do so within an hour of the first symptoms. The reason is cardiac arrhythmias: wildly erratic electrical activity of cardiac cells that impede the pumping action of the heart, halting flow of blood to the vital organs, including the brain. Multiple studies across many species, including humans, now document that heart victims with high levels of omega-3 fatty acids in the body have a drastically reduced risk of cardiac sudden death.

  Cardiologist Alexander Leaf of Harvard Medical School has performed landmark studies on omega-3s and sudden cardiac death. In a series of elegant experiments, Leaf and colleagues found a way to induce fatal cardiac arrhythmias in animals by abruptly closing off key coronary arteries, thus inducing a fatal heart attack. But animals pretreated with high levels of omega-3 fatty acids through dietary fish oil had far lower rates of sudden cardiac death following the induced, experimental heart attacks than did control animals. In another study, Leaf's group was able to rapidly stop what would have been an otherwise fatal arrhythmia through intravenous infusions of omega-3 fatty acids. Leaf and other investigators have also determined the biochemical mechanism underlying the antiarrhythmic effect of the omega-3 fatty acids.

All three of the common omega-3 fatty acids (EPA, DHA, and ALA) stabilize heart cells by affecting crucial membrane structures known as "ion channels" for the ions calcium, sodium, and potassium. The amount of these ions moving into and out of the cell through the ion channels is kept under tight control and determines the electrical activity of each heart cell on a microscopic level and the pumping power of the entire heart at a macroscopic level. All three common omega-3 fatty acids stabilize the cardiac muscle cell by regulating ion channels. They attach to a protein next to the ion channels, reducing the abnormal electrical activity in the cardiac muscle, and thus providing the body with natural protection against deadly cardiac arrhythmias.

The human data documenting the cardioprotective effects of omega-3 fatty acids have grown steadily over the past two decades. In the Physicians Health Study, an epidemiological study of 20,000 U.S. doctors, those who initially reported eating fish at least once a week were half as likely to succumb to a cardiac sudden death over the next decade as those who ate fish less than once a month. And in a British study, male heart attack survivors were asked to eat at least two weekly portions of fatty fish like salmon, trout, mackerel, herring, or sardines, while a control group maintained the medical establishment's recommended "heart-healthy" diet. After two years, fish eaters had a 29 percent lower risk of cardiac sudden death.

* *Reduced risk of heart attack.* Heart attacks occur when coronary arteries supplying oxygen-laden blood to the heart become blocked due to atherosclerosis or other causes, preventing sufficient oxygen from reaching a region of the heart. If the lack of oxygen (known as ischemia) continues for more than a few minutes, the affected heart cells die.

  Omega-3 oils reduce the risk of these potentially deadly cardiac events on a number of fronts. Known for their anti-inflammatory action throughout the body, the omega-3 fatty acids may reduce arterial inflammation, a condition associated with cardiac death. A 1997 study in the *New England Journal of Medicine* showed that men with a marker in their blood associated with severely inflamed arteries are three times more likely to suffer heart attack as men with normal arteries. Omega-3 fatty acids also fight the plaque that builds up on the inside of arteries by raising levels of HDL cholesterol, which counteracts the LDL cholesterol that forms plaque in the first place.

* *Reduced risk of blood clots.* These clots, which may block an already narrow or inflamed coronary artery, are formed in part by platelets clumping together. Aspirin, known to reduce the risk of heart attack, prevents platelets from sticking together, thereby reducing the chance of clot formation in coronary arteries. Omega-3 fatty acids have a similar effect on platelet stickiness.

Why Don't More Cardiologists Recommend Omega-3 Fatty Acids?

The 1999 Italian study published in the *Lancet* was definitive in demonstrating that omega-3s lower the risk of fatal and nonfatal heart attacks and stroke, while also reducing the rate of cardiac sudden death by 30 percent. Despite this and other impressive research findings, many cardiologists do not recommend increased fish consumption or omega-3 fatty acid supplements for their patients. Over the past several years, I have asked a number of cardiologists why they fail to make this recommendation. Many report being unaware of the scientific strength of the omega-3 studies in cardiology. This lack of awareness may be related to the fact that omega-3 essential fatty acids from fish oil are considered a food or an over-the-counter dietary supplement, and therefore no pharmaceutical company is promoting fish oil supplements to physicians.

Pharmaceutical companies may invest tens or even hundreds of millions of dollars in the development of a single patented new drug. The patent prevents anyone else from marketing their drug during its twenty-year patent life. Only totally new chemical structures or uses may be patented. Since the omega-3 fatty acids are natural substances, which have been described in the medical literature for decades, their chemical structures cannot be protected by patent and they are therefore unattractive to profit-seeking pharmaceutical companies. Once the prolonged process of Food and Drug Administration (FDA) approval is completed, huge marketing and public relations campaigns are aimed at doctors, and now the lay public, to increase sales of the medication. Without a corporate sponsor, the omega-3 fatty acids are likely to remain pharmaceutical orphans for the foreseeable future. As awareness of the health benefits of the omega-3s grows, perhaps the public itself will compel the medical profession to incorporate them into routine practice.

Metabolic Balance: Why Omega-3 Oils May Reduce Obesity and Ease the Symptoms of Diabetes

The dramatic increase in obesity over the past few decades has been the subject of endless debate, with pundits blaming everything from the sedentary service economy to the Big Mac. Why have Americans gained more weight more rapidly than ever before? Why are our children becoming increasingly obese? Reduced physical activity is clearly an important factor. One other emerging hypothesis is that the rise in obesity may be linked to a deficit of omega-3 fatty acids. The omega-3s, along with their molecular foils, the omega-6s, mediate many aspects of metabolism, including the level of sugar in the blood, as well as how we burn fat. The latest studies indicate that excessive omega-6 fatty acids may be partially responsible for irregularities in blood glucose, insulin, and energy production, resulting in obesity, diabetes, and other metabolic ills.

Keeping blood sugar in balance is one of our most vital physiological tasks. As we eat and digest our food, the body's basic fuel—glucose—enters and accumulates in the blood. Too much blood glucose is toxic, causing dehydration, multiple medical problems, and eventually coma and death. Too little blood glucose is tantamount to starvation; without basic nutrients, the body's organs, including the brain, will die. Thus, a major goal of metabolism is to hold the blood glucose level steady within a narrow range, providing a constant source of nourishment for our cells.

One cornerstone of this metabolic balance is the circulating hormone insulin, produced by pancreatic islet cells when blood sugar gets sufficiently high. When the system is healthy, insulin tells muscles to siphon glucose from the blood, providing the muscles with glucose for their energy needs, but also for short-term storage of glucose in the form of glycogen, a large polymer molecule composed of repeating units of glucose. Marathon runners rely on the glycogen in their muscles to sustain their energy. But when muscles are "insulin resistant"—they ignore insulin's signal—the system breaks down. Sugar, in the form of glucose meant to power the muscles, accumulates in the blood with toxic effects. The last stop on the pathway of insulin resistance is diabetes, a group of conditions in which the body either does not respond to insulin or manufactures no insulin at all.

Three Types of Diabetes

According to the National Diabetes Information Clearing-house, there are three main types of diabetes: insulin-dependent diabetes mellitus (IDDM) or Type I diabetes, noninsulin-dependent diabetes mellitus (NIDDM) or Type II diabetes, and gestational diabetes.

Insulin-Dependent Diabetes. Insulin-dependent diabetes is considered by many to be an autoimmune disease—one that results when the body's system for fighting infection (the immune system) turns against a part of the body. In diabetes, the immune system attacks the insulin-producing islet cells in the pancreas and destroys them. The pancreas then produces little or no insulin. Someone with IDDM needs daily injections of insulin to live. Scientists do not know exactly what causes the body's immune system to attack the islet cells, but they believe that both genetic factors and viruses are involved. IDDM accounts for about 5 to 10 percent of diagnosed diabetes in the United States.

IDDM develops most often in children and young adults, but the disorder can appear at any age. Symptoms usually develop over a short period, although islet cell destruction can begin months or even years earlier. Symptoms include increased thirst and urination, constant hunger, weight loss, blurred vision, and extreme tiredness. If IDDM is not diagnosed and treated with insulin, a person can lapse into a life-threatening coma.

Noninsulin-Dependent Diabetes. The most common form of diabetes is noninsulin-dependent diabetes. About 90 to 95 percent of people with diabetes have NIDDM. This form of diabetes usually develops in adults over the age of forty and is most common among adults over age fifty-five. About 80 percent of people with NIDDM are overweight. In NIDDM, the pancreas usually produces insulin, but for some reason, the body cannot respond to it effectively. (It is, in other words, insulin-resistant.) The result is the same as for IDDM: an unhealthy buildup of glucose in the blood and an inability of the body to make efficient use of its main source of fuel. The symptoms of NIDDM develop gradually and are not as noticeable as in IDDM. Symptoms include feeling tired or ill, frequent urination (especially at night), unusual thirst, weight loss, blurred vision, frequent infections, and slow healing of sores.

Gestational Diabetes. Gestational diabetes develops or is discovered during pregnancy. It usually disappears when the pregnancy is over, but women who have had gestational diabetes have a far greater risk of developing diabetes later in their lives.

Now a series of studies from Australia show that excess omega-6 fatty acids along with a deficit of the omega-3s may contribute to insulin resistance, and omega-3 fatty acid supplements may decrease insulin resistance or even prevent the development of diabetes. The news is of great importance for public health, as diabetes is a huge cause of death and disability.

Piqued by finding the Inuit Eskimos have surprisingly low rates of adult-onset diabetes, a team from Australia's Garvan Institute of Medical Research fed laboratory rats a diet rich in saturated and unsaturated fats from plant and animal sources. The rats soon developed insulin resistance, the team reported in the journal *Science*. But when the researchers fed the rats with omega-3 fatty acids from fish oil, the resistance problem disappeared.

Picking up where the Garvan team left off, Dr. Leonard Storlien, then of the University of Sydney, found that the omega-3 effect could be documented in human diabetics as well. In one study, he found that diets rich in long-chain omega-3 fatty acids could significantly overcome insulin resistance in diabetics. In a subsequent Storlien study, researchers biopsied skeletal muscle from twenty men and seven women between the ages of fifty and sixty-five; all were nondiabetic and undergoing coronary bypass surgery. Nonetheless, the researchers correlated fatty acids in the cell membranes with each patient's sensitivity to insulin. In general, they reported in the *New England Journal of Medicine*, the more saturated fatty acids present, the more resistant a patient proved to insulin.

In his most recent research, Storlien (now at the University of Wollon-gong in Australia) assigned fifty-five patients with non-insulin-dependent diabetes mellitus to either a fat-modified diet (high in monounsaturated fat and omega-3s and low in omega-6) or a high-carbohydrate diet. After one year, Storlien found, insulin sensitivity was significantly higher in people on the high omega-3 diet than those on the high-carbohydrate diet.

According to Storlien, the low omega-6 to omega-3 ratio was also key to modulating obesity in those he studied as well. This may explain why Israeli Jews suffer more diabetes and obesity than Americans. Although the typical Israeli diet is lower in calories and fat, Israelis also consume more omega-6 oils than any other population in the world. People with muscles low in omega-3 fatty acids and high in omega-6 are more likely to be not only insulin resistant but also obese.

Other research supports the link between omega-3s and weight loss. Baillie and colleagues at the University of Texas in Austin showed that mice raised on fish oil (omega-3) instead of corn oil (omega-6) were 25 percent leaner, even when their caloric intake was the same. The mechanism responsible for the weight loss observed with omega-3s is hypothesized to be thermogenesis (literally "heat generating"). When fed a high-omega-3 diet, the body uses more energy to burn the same number of calories, resulting in weight loss and the generation of excess heat. In animal models, and possibly people, the omega-3 fatty acids caused a loss of fat in specific regions of the body. DHA and EPA achieve this by fitting into a specific receptor inside the cell at the nucleus, called peroxisomal proliferator activated receptors (PPARs). Only recently discovered, PPARs show that omega-3s directly activate the expression of the genes controlling fat metabolism. The fact that omega-3s can directly alter gene expression demonstrates how central the essential fatty acids are for health.

What is true for the rat may be true for humans. In clinical studies of omega-3 fatty acids, weight gain did not occur. In fact, some people lost weight. This observation is consistent with a study published in 1991, which showed that Japanese men who migrated to the United States were significantly more obese than their counterparts who remained in Japan. The major difference in these two groups was a marked drop in fish (omega-3) consumption in the Japanese men who left their native country. If omega-3 fatty acids are associated with weight loss or prevent the development of obesity and diabetes, this could have powerful implications for adults and children. More research is needed to clarify the precise roles of omega-3s in energy and metabolism.

Omega-3 Fatty Acids and Immunity

Rheumatoid arthritis, Crohn's disease, lupus, and asthma are a group of illnesses with widely differing symptoms and locations in the body. Nonetheless, all seem to involve the omega-6 and omega-3 fatty acids and aspects of the immune system and inflammation that have somehow gone out of control.

In yin-yang fashion, the balance of omega-6 to omega-3 fatty acids strongly influences the immune system. They exert this power through their central role in the physiological process of inflammation, essential for healing injured or infected tissue by engulfing and destroying invading organisms before they can overrun our bodies and cause illness or death.

When we take a fall and cut our knee or when we come down with a cold, inflammation is our body's first response to danger. Chemically recognizing the injury or infection almost immediately, our body dispatches different types of cells to the affected area. If there is an injury with bleeding, platelets will detect damaged tissue and aggregate to begin the process of blood clotting. Different types of white blood cells will be attracted to the area by local chemical signals released by the damaged or infected tissue. The white blood cells, platelets, and other cell types have begun the inflammatory process. This causes the characteristic signs and symptoms of inflammation in the affected area: redness, warmth, swelling, and pain.

These clinical signs result from the tremendous activity that is occurring on the biochemical and microscopic level. The white blood cells, frontline soldiers of the immune system, surround the invading organisms. Large, specialized white blood cells called macrophages, attracted by the chemicals of inflammation, enter the area and engulf the bacteria or virus. The invaders, captured in tiny sacs within the macrophage, are ultimately destroyed by chemical bioweapons, including free radicals.

In some people, a genetic vulnerability, an unusual response to an infection or some other factor causes the inflammatory or immune response to be overactive. If this process persists and is severe enough, autoimmune disorders may be the result. When the body's inflammation-related immune response attacks the joints, genetically predisposed victims may suffer the chronic pain and disfigurement of rheumatoid arthritis. Unleashed in the respiratory tract, a deregulated immune response may cause allergies and asthma. Gone awry in the gastrointestinal system, immune dysfunction can set the stage for inflammatory bowel diseases such as Crohn's disease and ulcerative colitis.

Omega-6 and omega-3 fatty acids have a major role in the immune response and in inflammation. The omega-6 eicosanoids produce a strong inflammatory response; when balanced with the mildly inflammatory omega-3 eicosanoids, the strength of the inflammatory response is appropriate. But if omega-6 eicosanoids predominate, then the inflammatory response can be excessive for any given situation. A chronically overactive inflammatory response may lead to disease in many different organ systems.

The inflammatory response and the eicosanoids also play a role in mood disorders and the brain. Since the body uses the same or similar biochemical processes in different organ systems, it is hardly surprising to learn that eicosanoids can also be found in the brain. A detailed knowledge of eicosanoids in the brain is needed, but recent research associates depression with the same type of essential fatty acid imbalance found at the root of autoimmune disease. (A detailed discussion is found in chapter 6.)

Researchers first connected essential fatty acid imbalance to autoimmune disease in the 1970s, when they realized that Greenland Eskimos consuming diets high in omega-3 fatty acids rarely suffered from arthritis, asthma, or other disorders associated with excess inflammation. Since that time, a body of research has begun exploring the connection in depth. High levels of omega-6 are almost always associated with inflammation; omega-3 applies the brakes.

Guided by the biochemistry, researchers have found omega-3 fatty acids helpful in the treatment of inflammation-related immune disease across the board. Some areas of focus include the following:

- *Rheumatoid arthritis*, an inflammatory joint disease. In a series of studies over the past decade the omega-3 fatty acids have been observed consistently to reduce swelling, irritation, and pain associated with rheumatoid arthritis. In more than a dozen studies conducted during the 1990s, rheumatoid arthritis patients taking omega-3 fatty acid supplements experienced less stiffness and fewer tender and swollen joints than they had without taking the capsules. In some instances, patients were able to taper or discontinue their use of anti-inflammatory medication, including aspirin, ibuprofen, and other so-called nonsteroidal anti-inflammatory drugs, which can cause bleeding and gastrointestinal pain. In a recent Australian study, rheumatoid arthritis patients already receiving conventional therapies were given supplements of fish or olive oil. After twelve weeks, the fish oil group showed marked benefit—and accompanying the clinical improvement was a 30 percent reduction in levels of highly inflammatory omega-6–derived eicosanoids. The olive oil group showed no improvement.

In 2000, Curtis and colleagues at Cardiff University, Wales, made a major discovery by showing that omega-3s can inhibit cox-2, a pro-inflammatory enzyme, blocked by such new anti-arthritis drugs as Celebrex. The omega-3s also appear to decrease cartilage damage resulting from attack by other enzymes.

• *Crohn's disease*, a debilitating inflammation of the gastrointestinal tract, with symptoms of cramping, nausea, diarrhea, and bleeding as well as weakness, weight loss, and depression. Crohn's disease can affect every organ system, and cases exist where the gastrointestinal symptoms are mild while a multitude of other possible symptoms erupt. The presence of baffling and inconsistent symptoms in Crohn's disease sometimes leads to years of misdiagnosis and inappropriate treatment. Known for cycles of relapse and remission, Crohn's disease has long eluded safe and reliably effective treatments to prolong the symptom-free periods. But an Italian study published several years ago in the *New England Journal of Medicine* shows that omega-3 fatty acids may offer the possibility of an alternative or adjunctive treatment. Studying 78 patients in remission from Crohn's disease, the researchers gave half the group 2.7 grams of EPA and DHA in capsule form each day while the other half received a placebo. After a year, 59 percent of the fish oil group remained in remission, as opposed to just 26 percent of the placebo group.

A St. Louis study, meanwhile, found that supplements of omega-3 fatty acids were beneficial to patients with another inflammatory bowel disease—ulcerative colitis, characterized by inflammation of the large intestine that sometimes is so severe it can be fatal. Patients using omega-3 fatty acid supplements were able to halve their dosage of corticosteroid drugs. Corticosteroids, such as prednisone and cortisone, are associated with immune suppression, weight gain, mood changes, and other severe side effects. The biochemical mechanism or mechanisms by which omega-3 fatty acids control inflammatory bowel disease are unclear, but it seems distinct from many of the medication regimens patients currently receive. Whether used alone in mild forms of inflammatory bowel disease, or in combination with other, more conventional agents in moderate or severe forms of inflammatory bowel disease, the omega-3 fatty acids merit further study.

- *Systemic lupus erythematosus*, an immune disorder that can ravage the body, attacking organs from kidney to brain. In numerous studies of animals with lupus-like illness or humans with actual lupus, omega-3 fatty acids have reduced inflammation, kidney problems, and mortality. A New Zealand study of mice found the disease slowed remarkably when omega-3 oils were added to the diet. In a recent U.S. study, patients with active lupus showed significant improvement on supplements of omega-3 oils. In a study in India, investigators found that omega-3 fatty acids could cause an actual remission from lupus. While it may be unlikely that most patients with lupus could replace their conventional anti-inflammatory drugs with omega-3 fatty acids, there may be a place for using the omega-3s as adjuncts. More research is needed.

- *Asthma*, a recurrent condition where the small airways in the lung become suddenly constricted. Asthma is marked by wheezing, breathlessness, and tightness of the chest, which can be fatal if severe and untreated. Like depression, cancer, and so many other modern disorders, it is inexplicably on the rise, particularly in children. Whether or not lack of omega-3 fatty acids is a factor in this increase, as some investigators suggest, evidence suggests omega-3 fatty acids may be part of the cure. Among 468 Australian children, those who ate one serving of omega-3-rich fish per week were 25 percent less likely to have asthma than those who did not eat those fish, according to a study in the *Medical Journal of Australia*. The study found that for every four children prone to asthma, two would not get it if they included oily fish in their diet. And in a recent one-year study done in France, asthmatics who took about 1 gram of omega-3 fatty acids per day had greater improvements in lung capacity than controls did.

Preliminary studies suggest that omega-3 fatty acids may provide relief from a range of other types of inflammatory disorders, including menstrual cramps, migraine, and the gum disease gingivitis. Individuals with lupus or other inflammatory disorders often experience dramatic, near-immediate relief from corticosteroid therapy. However, the long-term risk and the adverse effects make chronic corticosteroid therapy problematic. If proved effective, omega-3 fatty acids might well be welcome adjuncts, or possibly substitutes for some, in the treatment of those with a range of immune-related inflammatory disorders.

Cancer and Cell Death

Cancer, a result of unchecked proliferation of abnormal cells in the body's tissues or bloodstream, can strike any organ system in the body. In individuals with cancer there is a lessened ability to identify and destroy cells that have turned cancerous, an ability that functions well in those without the disease. Recent studies suggest that omega-6 fatty acids, which accelerate cell growth, may also promote cancerous growth. As in other biochemical processes described earlier, the omega-3s have actions that oppose omega-6 activity. Increased consumption of omega-3s might keep accelerated cell growth, as seen in cancer, contained.

Cancer is a complex illness, with many factors contributing to its genesis, malignant growth, and cure. The balance of omega-3 and omega-6 fatty acids appears to be relevant for certain tumors, but further research is needed to characterize fully the role of the fatty acids in cancer.

One tantalizing clue to this role came when cancer researchers Leonard Sauer and Robert Daucy sought to learn why tumors grew faster in starving laboratory rats, when the opposite should have been true. Indeed, since cancer is largely about cell growth, it stands to reason that starvation would slow cancer, not rev it up. But looking more closely, the scientists found that conditions of famine shifted rats into an altered, hyperactive metabolic state. Responding to the problem, the rats released their fat stores to the bloodstream, raising the fat level some five times higher than normal. Perhaps feasting on the fat molecules, tumors grew rapidly, with rates of growth slowing only when the normal food supply was restored.

The observation caused the team to step back and wonder: would tumor growth vary depending on the type of fat, or did all fats affect cancers in exactly the same way? Exposing tumors to different types of fat, they found that by far the most carcinogenic (cancer-producing) was linoleic acid, an omega-6. (Remarkably, omega-6 fatty acids increased tumor growth far more than did the saturated fats.) By contrast, when tumors were exposed to omega-3 fatty acids, their rate of growth slowed. These findings suggest some role for the competing omega-3 and omega-6 eicosanoid pathways in at least some cancers.

A large-scale epidemiological study has recently suggested that omega-3 fatty acids may be therapeutic for human cancer patients too. Following the same test group of 605 he studied in the Lyon Diet Heart Study, Michel de Lorgeril found that those consuming high levels of omega-3 fatty acids in their diet were 56 percent less likely to get cancer and 61 percent less likely to die of it than controls.

Omega-3 fatty acids have been shown possibly to prevent cancer and slow cancerous growth in other studies too. Breast tumor production is less aggressive in lab animals fed fish oils. Other evidence suggests that the effect may hold true for humans. Scientists at the University of California at Los Angeles, for instance, placed twenty-five women with breast cancer on a low-fat diet that included 3 grams of omega-3 fatty acids a day—the amount in two 3-ounce servings of mackerel or salmon. Biopsies after three months showed that the ratio of omega-3 fatty acids to other fatty acids in the fatty portion of the women's breast tissue went up significantly. That made sense, because the composition of body fat tends to reflect fat in the diet. Of interest was the finding that the proportion of omega-3 fatty acids also increased in other fatty tissues in the women's bodies, but to a smaller degree, indicating that fish oil might play a special role in the breast. The findings are relevant in light of French research showing that women with low levels of omega-3 molecules in breast tissue are five times more likely than controls to develop breast cancer.

Although omega-3 fatty acids may lower risk for cancer, they are unlikely to be the primary therapy for any form of cancer. Much, much more research needs to be done to explore these connections. Nonetheless, there is reason to believe they may prove valuable as health-promoting adjuncts to chemotherapy, radiation, and surgery. Already this role seems possible. In one impressive study, cancer patients recovering from surgery and placed on omega-3 fatty acids had 50 percent fewer infections, lower levels of triglycerides, and better kidney and liver function than controls. In experiments with mice, omega-3 supplements rendered chemotherapy both more effective and less toxic.

Scientists still do not know why omega-3 fatty acids may reduce risk for cancer and slow its growth and whether these findings extend beyond the animal models. The most obvious hypothesis involves a change in the balance of omega-3 versus omega-6 eicosanoids, which somehow alters either the tumor or the body's response to it. Pinpointing the precise role of omega-3 fatty acids in cancer may prove essential to understanding the basic biochemistry needed to develop future cures. Even at this point, however, there is a great deal of evidence for the beneficial role of omega-3s in many of our body systems—enough to illustrate why we have chosen to call this chapter, and the omega-3 oils themselves, the Wellness Molecules.

5

Pregnancy and Postpartum Depression

✍ In the moment of fertilization, the egg and sperm join to form a single cell, the zygote. In the first hours and days of life, the zygote will divide again and again, ultimately giving rise to the specialized cells and organs of the baby. As the cells and organs differentiate, taking on final form, their nutritional requirements will come to differ as well.

The developing brain in particular has a huge and absolute requirement for energy in the form of oxygen and glucose, and for structural molecules, including fatty acids of the omega-6 and omega-3 class. As the fetal brain grows from a few hundred cells to billions of neurons and supporting cells, it draws these essential elements from the blood. The bloodstream ultimately touches every brain cell—like all cells—through tiny blood vessels called capillaries, which permeate the entire tissue.

The substances that flow through the fetal bloodstream originate with the mother. Inhaled oxygen and nutrients extracted from food eaten by the mother flow through her bloodstream and travel to the placenta. There, the bloodstreams of mother and baby come in intimate contact, ultimately transferring the vital nutrients and oxygen to the fetus developing in the womb via the umbilical cord. When maternal blood is rich in oxygen and appropriate nutrients, the unborn child can thrive. But thousands of research studies document the consequences when maternal blood is deficient in some nutrients. Maternal deficit of folic acid, for instance, can result in babies with spina bifida (a neural tube deficit where the spinal column fails to close). Smoking mothers put the developing fetus at risk for premature birth and, later, learning problems, due either to the reduced oxygen or to the carbon monoxide or other toxins within the cigarette smoke. Even moderate amounts of alcohol during the early months of pregnancy can cause fetal alcohol syndrome, notable for mental retardation and developmental delays.

As a society, we have tried to address these problems. Supplements of folic acid and other vitamins offer some protection against some fetal malformations, such as neural tube defects. Restaurants carry signs warning against ingesting alcohol during pregnancy. And for those who receive regular prenatal care, attention to a balanced diet throughout pregnancy has become a given.

But despite the new vigilance, one nutrient group has fallen through the cracks: the omega-3 oils, necessary not just for evolution of the human brain but also for its growth in the womb. Both old and new research indicates that a lack of omega-3s during gestation may impair development of the visual system and may compromise future intelligence.

Since essential fatty acids cannot be manufactured by the human body, the fetus acquires all omega-3s from the mother's bloodstream, and ultimately from her diet and the stores of EPA and DHA in her tissues. Imagine a scenario in which the mother is partially depleted of omega-3 fatty acids. Since omega-3 fatty acids are actively transported to the developing baby, EPA and DHA will be siphoned off from the mother to meet the high demand of the baby's brain and body development. If there is just enough for the baby, fetal development can proceed normally.

The outcome for the mother in this situation is less certain. Depleted of omega-3 fatty acids, the pregnant and then postpartum woman may experience a host of health problems. The situation is possibly worse in the case of the pregnant woman very depleted of omega-3s. In this case, neither the mother nor the developing baby will have adequate levels of omega-3 oils, laying the groundwork for a host of documented health consequences.

Omega-3 Fatty Acid Depletion in Postpartum Women

- Omega-3s are preferentially transported to the developing fetus.
- Depletion in pregnancy and in postpartum women is well documented.
- Omega-3 loss is greater in multiple births.
- Omega-3 loss may normalize after about one year.
- DHA loss through lactation is detectable within eight weeks postpartum.
- The degree of omega-3 loss is largely dependent on diet.

High-Risk Pregnancy

Omega-3 deficit during pregnancy delivers a devastating double blow: it compromises the future integrity of the baby's brain and possibly general health and may affect the mother's current and future health as well as perhaps putting the pregnancy itself at risk.

Numerous studies in the past decade have traced omega-3 deficit to one of pregnancy's potentially most life-threatening problems, preeclampsia and eclampsia. The precise cause of these disorders remains obscure. The symptoms of eclampsia include high blood pressure, headache, blurred vision, breathlessness, nausea, swelling, pain in the upper right quadrant of the abdomen, and epilepsy-like convulsions. Untreated, it can cause permanent kidney and liver damage as well as maternal and fetal death. Although other biochemical processes are likely involved, the evidence points to a possible role for the omega-3s. Pregnant women with preeclampsia have lower levels of EPA and DHA (the long-chain omega-3s) than pregnant women without preeclampsia.

According to a 1999 report in the *Journal of the American Medical Association*, women with preeclampsia have significantly lower levels of the omega-3–derived eicosanoid prostacyclin, a vasodilator, and are therefore far more prone to constriction of the blood vessels and a decreased flow of blood through the placenta. In a balancing act characteristic of the essential fatty acids, omega-3s increase levels of prostacyclin, while their antagonists, the omega-6 oils, increase levels of opposing eicosanoids, thromboxane A2 and B2, blood vessel constrictors. Consistent with what is known about the eicosanoids, the evidence suggests that omega-3 supplements may lower the chances of developing preeclampsia in the first place. It is important to note that no study has ever administered more than 3.5 grams per day of EPA and DHA together to a pregnant woman.

Omega-3 deficit has also been associated with low birthweight and premature birth, the largest cause of infant mortality. In contrast, newborns in the Faroe Islands, located in the North Atlantic between Norway and Iceland, have the highest average birthweight out of thirty-three geographic regions sampled in a recent study. Scientists have hypothesized that this is due to a diet rich in fish and high levels of EPA, thought to markedly alter quantities of eicosanoids needed for labor and delivery. Specifically, they postulate that increased omega-3 gives rise to increased levels of prostacyclins, which relax uterine muscles and thus delay the onset of labor while at the same time reducing relative levels of specific omega-6–derived prostaglandins, which stimulate labor and delivery.

Testing this notion, scientists compared length of pregnancy for sixty-two new mothers at Landssjukrahusid, the main hospital in the Faroe Islands, with thirty-seven counterparts at Aarhus University Hospital in Denmark. At first glance, the omega-3 effect seemed relatively minor, with pregnancies lasting just two days longer on average for Faroese women than for the Danes. The surprise came when scientists looked at the Danish women alone. Within this population, women with the highest omega-3 to omega-6 ratios gave birth on average 5.7 days later than those with ratios about 20 percent lower. The researchers attribute the phenomenon to a threshold effect: when a woman is adequately nourished, extra omega-3s do not make a difference, but when there is a deficit, premature birth and correspondingly lower birthweights may result.

Can supplements of omega-3 oils during pregnancy directly lower the risk of premature birth? Follow-up research on Danish women shows they may. To test the possibility, Sjurdur Olsen of the Institute of Epidemiology and Social Medicine, University of Aarhus, worked with 533 patients at a midwife clinic. During the third trimester of pregnancy, one group received fish oil capsules (a source of omega-3 fatty acids), another group received capsules of olive oil (mainly a source of omega-9 and some omega-6 fatty acids), and a third received no oil at all. While just 14 percent of the women taking fish oil supplements delivered early, percentages increased to 16 percent for the group taking no oil and to a statistically significant 24 percent for those on olive oil. As expected, women on fish oil supplements had longer pregnancies and higher-birthweight babies as well. Says Olson, "Fish oil supplementation in late pregnancy seems to delay delivery, without affecting the continued growth of the fetus. Our findings suggest an easy and cheap intervention to prevent pre-term delivery."

Omega-3 Fatty Acids: Critical in Brain Development

- Omega-3 fatty acids are concentrated in breast milk (but not in U.S. formula).
- DHA and EPA are abundant essential lipids in the brain.
- EPA is converted into the powerful signaling molecules, the eicosanoids, which are crucial to brain function.
- DHA and EPA are incorporated into neuronal membranes.
- DHA and EPA may produce a more "fluid" membrane.

- DHA improves cognitive and visual function in infants (which explains the breast-fed versus bottle-fed disparity).
- Premature babies are the most vulnerable to omega-3 deficiency.
- Omega-3 fatty acids are depleted in the U.S. diet.

Brain Building

Since omega-3s appear so essential to the evolution of the human brain, it is hardly surprising that we require them for building each individual brain from the earliest days in the womb. Yet developmental science considered essential fatty acids of marginal importance until the early 1960s, when the first signs of clinical deficiency became apparent in infants fed skim milk formula. The syndrome, marked by deficits in omega-6 and omega-3, included skin lesions; decreased skin pigmentation; loss of muscle tone; disordered functioning of the kidney, lung, and liver; and increased susceptibility to infection. The essential fatty acid deficiency syndrome could be reversed with supplements of linoleic acid (LA), an omega-6 oil.

Researchers recognized more insidious (and less reversible) problems stemming from omega-3 deficit alone. In species from rats to monkeys to humans, restriction of omega-3s during pregnancy and breast-feeding was associated with poorer, less developed visual skills and learning problems. In rhesus monkeys, visual abnormalities resulting from omega-3 deficit could not be reversed, even when omega-3 oils were supplied in quantity later in life.

Increasingly sophisticated analysis of brain composition and diet strengthened the argument that omega-3 fatty acid deficit was the cause. Across a range of mammalian species, studies linked reduced dietary intake of essential fatty acids to reduced brain levels of arachidonic acid (AA, from the omega-6 group) and DHA, from the omega-3 group. Even in lower species, AA and DHA, the long-chained versions of the essential fatty acids, are needed in equal proportion for efficient functioning of the visual system and the brain.

But humans are in a different league. Without large amounts of DHA, the long-chain omega-3 commonly found in fish, we might not have evolved at all. And a significant body of evidence now points to the impact when a deficiency of DHA occurs during critical periods of development for the brain. The strongest studies focus on the last three months of gestation and the first year of life—the developmental window during which the brain and retina are developing the most rapidly and most avidly accumulate DHA and associated visual and cognitive skills.

Because it is difficult to assess a baby in the womb, researchers have homed in on premature babies, which are developmentally comparable to babies in the last trimester of intrauterine life. Working with premature newborns in Dallas, Texas, and Santiago, Chile, a team led by Ricardo Uauy of the Universidad de Chile measured the impact of supplements comprised either of corn oil (LA, omega-6) or soy oil mixed with fish oil (EPA and DHA). Testing the composition of the blood at thirty-six and then fifty-seven weeks after conception, the scientists found that the babies given fish oil had markedly greater levels of DHA. Differences between the two groups were accentuated with time.

Fatty acid measurements in the blood were associated with striking functional differences between the two groups. At fifty-seven weeks after conception, the premature babies fed corn oil had immature visual systems and poorer visual skills while the premature babies fed fish oil were virtually identical to healthy, full-term, breast-fed infants of comparable gestational age. The researchers also observed that babies fed corn oil had immature sleep patterns, a sign of developmental delay, while those on the fish oil had sleep patterns similar to those of full-term babies.

Still more evidence comes from comparisons of breast- versus bottle-fed babies, since human milk contains high levels of DHA and formula does not. Literally hundreds of studies document the advantages of breast-feeding for the baby, pointing to lower risk for infectious diseases, calmer dispositions, and higher IQ, among other facts. Although most of the advantages of breast-feeding appear to be due to the presence of omega-3s, it is important to remember that breast-feeding provides potential developmental benefits other than nutritional: increased amounts of physical contact and maternal attention. One team compared a group of prematurely born infants bottle-fed breast milk to a set of prematurely born infants fed formula; when tested for IQ at age eight, the breast milk group scored on average 8.3 points higher than the group given cow's milk-based formula.

More recently, researchers reported on 526 full-term Dutch infants born between 1975 and 1979 and then followed for nine years. The 135 breast-fed infants in that study had significantly lower rates of neurological dysfunction than the rest of the group, which was fed on cow-milk-based formula alone. Another study shows that breast-fed babies are more developmentally advanced as early as two days after birth. Some women cannot breast-feed their babies, for a variety of reasons. Nevertheless, with close and intimate contact with the mother, along with omega-3–supplemented formulas, bottle-fed babies should be able to match the omega-3–facilitated brain and visual system development of breast-fed babies.

Eating for Two

Given the evidence, it seems wise to consider ways of delivering more omega-3s to unborn children and, later, to infants, providing them with nutrients historically required by the brain. The best strategy is altering maternal nutrition through diet and using selected omega-3 supplements before, during, and after pregnancy and birth. There may be a role for high-quality supplements, since eating excessive amounts of certain types of fish puts the mother and baby at risk for toxicity from a range of poisonous substances from mercury to organic chemical pollutants. Babies are particularly susceptible to the neurotoxic (literally "brain poisoning") effects of mercury and other contaminants. The Omega-3 Renewal Plan at the end of this book describes the pros and cons of fish versus supplements in more detail.

Regardless of diet, mature human milk contains roughly 50 percent fat, a requirement not only for the energy required to fuel the tremendous growth rate of newborn infants, but also for completing the structural development of the brain. The proportion of DHA and other omega-3 fatty acids in milk fat, however, varies widely from population to population. In study after study, researchers have found that the DHA content of mother's milk depends to a large degree on the types and quantities of foods consumed. The "hind" milk at the end of a feeding contains more fat and, therefore, more omega-3s than the milk earlier in the feeding.

Scientists from the Dalian Medical University in China and Oregon Health Sciences University in Portland joined forces to study 146 lactating women from five diverse regions of China: marine (coastal), rural (farming), pastoral (tending herds), and two urban areas. The women from all five regions consumed similar quantities of calories and carbohydrate, but their fat and fish consumption varied widely. As expected, women from the marine region ate the greatest amount of seafood—about 136 grams, or nearly 5 ounces, a day. The urban women, who came from coastal cities, consumed significant quantities as well. For pastoral and rural women, seafood consumption was negligible.

Differences in diet were reflected in the composition of the milk. In the marine region, DHA was 2.78 percent of the milk fat, compared to 0.88 percent and 0.82 percent for the two urban populations, 0.68 percent for the rural region and 0.44 percent for the pastoral region. Studies of Inuit Eskimos as well as Malaysian, Dominican, and Nigerian women, all coastal populations, have shown similar results. Compare this to the distressingly low range of between 0.05 percent and 0.59 percent in the United States and Britain.

Other studies not only examined the dietary intake of omega-3 fatty acids but also looked at links between maternal omega-3 stores and supplies available for the baby's developing brain. In an international study of women from the Netherlands, Hungary, Finland, England, and Ecuador, researchers drew blood from a test group of mothers at eighteen weeks, twenty-two weeks, and thirty-two weeks after conception. Shortly after the mothers gave birth, the researchers drew more blood from them and, to measure the baby's status, samples were taken from the umbilical cord.

The findings were fascinating. Although the dietary intake of maternal fatty acids remained fairly constant, the levels measured in the blood fell throughout pregnancy across all the groups, most likely indicating increased uptake of maternal omega-3 fatty acid stores by the fetus over time. Moreover, maternal and infant omega-3 levels were tightly linked within each population. Finnish mothers and infants had the highest levels and Hungarians the lowest. Especially pertinent was the discovery that small increases in maternal omega-3 were most profoundly reflected in Hungarian infants, who had lower supplies than other groups in the first place. The implication is that when maternal omega-3 is low, supplemental omega-3 fatty acids appear to be preferentially taken up by the fetus.

There is further evidence linking omega-3 in the newborn's diet directly to the baby's later cognitive abilities. Scientists at the University of Dundee in Great Britain studied forty-four infants born at full term; twenty-one received formula supplemented with omega-3 fatty acids from birth through four months of age, and twenty-three received formula without the supplement. When the infants reached ten months of age, the researchers tested each with a three-step problem: retrieving a toy from behind three separate barriers—a block of foam, a blue cloth, and a brown cover. Both groups of infants scored similarly on the first two steps, but babies on the DHA supplement scored significantly higher than their counterparts when it came to completing step three, suggesting that DHA supplements might have enhanced their ability to negotiate this sophisticated cognitive task.

P. Willets, head of the team, notes that three-step problems involve memory and attention, factors that might have been heightened by the DHA. Infants who fail the barrier and cloth steps, for instance, may fail to retrieve the toy because they forget the final goal or ignore it as a result of being distracted. Providing a possible explanation, Willets suggests that accumulation of DHA in nerve cell membranes speeds up information pro-cessing, making infants with the supplement more efficient. An-other explanation may be that DHA affects the brain structures involved in disengagement, which is the process of releasing at-tention from a stimulus. The longer it takes to turn attention from one element to the next, the longer the problem solving will take. The findings are important, says Willets, because higher scores are related to higher IQ in childhood. "The scores suggest that benefits will persist beyond the period during which the infants received the supplemented formula."

The Formula Debate

While breast-feeding mothers can provide their babies with more omega-3s after birth by changes in diet or through omega-3 supplements, others must rely on the content of the few infant formula brands currently available. Yet despite the seemingly overwhelming evidence, the U.S. government and the formula industry have taken a dubious wait-and-see attitude about ap-proving infant formula supplemented with DHA. After all, skep-tics say, breast milk contains many other nutrients that could affect cognitive ability. In addition, breast-feeding mothers in the United States tend to be relatively well educated and finan-cially secure, both variables that could positively influence an infant's cognitive and learning capacity. It is hard to eliminate such effects, even in well-controlled studies. The situation is complicated by the presence of DHA in neural membranes throughout the brain. If widespread depletion exists, it would af-fect not just one element of intelligence and cognition but many—from memory and spatial skills to attention and learning. Teasing those factors apart is intricate, particularly in preverbal infant research subjects.

For years, skeptics argued that babies were making DHA from alpha-linolenic acid (ALA), the shorter-chain omega-3 molecule also present in breast milk and to a small degree in infant for-mula. But the latest evidence shows that this may not be the case.

Infants, like adults, have a limited ability to convert ALA to DHA. To boost brain growth and visual skill, abundant amounts of DHA (balanced with the omega-6 arachidonic acid) are best.

Although all the facts are not yet in, advocates say that formula with omega-3 levels comparable to that of an ideal breast milk would be the wisest course. Most nations of the world agree. DHA for babies is recommended by the World Health Organization and the Commission of the European Community. Drawn from fish, omega-3-enriched eggs, and algae, infant formula with DHA is available throughout Europe and Asia, in some sixty countries worldwide.

Yet in the United States, the Food and Drug Administration (FDA) says it does not have enough evidence to require omega-3 supplements in formula. Many DHA advocates believe that economic forces, including the hit to corporate profits of adding DHA to each serving of formula, are what is really at stake.

I believe the evidence overwhelmingly supports supplementing infant formula with long-chain omega-3 fatty acids, crucial building blocks of the brain. The debate over omega-3 oils in formula seems in some ways like the debate over the relationship between cigarettes and cancer. For decades, the cigarette industry claimed there were not enough data to prove smoking dangerous or addictive. But how many studies are enough? For decades, virtually every objective expert, the U.S. courts, and now some cigarette manufacturers themselves say the data showing the dangers of tobacco smoke are overwhelming. A review of the scientific literature suggests a comparable situation in the infant formula business, although in the case of infant formula, with a few exceptions, the disturbing truth has been largely ignored by the press (see Table 5–1).

Postpartum Depression

Lack of omega-3 oils can damage the health of mothers after birth too. Depleted of these essential lipids by the fetus, who receives them preferentially if there is any shortage, the mother is presumably at risk for any of the illnesses related to an omega-3 deficit.

Table 5–1: Composition of Human Breast Milk and U.S. Infant Formula

Breast Milk or Infant Formula Source	Ratio of Omega-6 to Long-Chain Omega-3 *
Breast milk (Inuit, Canada)	3.8 to 1
Breast milk, coastal (marine China)	7.1 to 1
Breast milk (Japan)	9.9 to 1
Breast milk, urban (China)	24.4 to 1
Breast milk, rural (inland China)	28.2 to 1
Breast milk (United States, Study 2)	67.4 to 1
Breast milk (United States, Study 1)	175 to 1
Mead Johnson ProSobee, with iron, ready to feed	No long-chain omega-3 fatty acids
Wyeth-Ayerst, SMA, low iron, ready to feed	No long-chain omega-3 fatty acids
Carnation Good Start, with iron, ready to feed	No long-chain omega-3 fatty acids
Ross, Similac, with iron, ready to feed	No long-chain omega-3 fatty acids

* These figures did not include the short chain omega-3 ALA, which would tend to reduce the omega-6 to omega-3 ratio.

But the most notable consequence may be postpartum depression. Blood levels of omega-3 fatty acids decrease during the latter stages of pregnancy and stay low, particularly in lactating women. Since circulating long-chain omega-3s are so important in cell-signaling pathways, and are integral to the structure and function of many brain systems, including those neural systems mediating mood and emotion, it makes sense that depletion might be a major cause of postpartum blues, as well as the more serious condition of postpartum major depression.

To test the notion that omega-3 fatty acid depletion is related at least in part to postpartum psychiatric disorder, Dr. Joseph R. Hibbeln of the National Institute on Alcohol Abuse and Alcoholism in Bethesda, Maryland, conducted a simple and elegant epidemiological study of fish consumption and the corresponding risk for postpartum depression in countries around the world. His extraordinary findings show a strong and direct association: when fish consumption rises, postpartum depression falls. Across the board, nations with high levels of fish consumption (Japan, Hong Kong, Sweden, and Chile) had the lowest levels of postpartum depression, and nations with low levels of fish consumption (Brazil, South Africa, West Germany, Saudi Arabia) had the highest rates of postpartum depression.

Many researchers and clinicians are suggesting fighting postpartum depression with omega-3 fatty acid supplements during pregnancy and after birth. To test the concept in a preliminary trial, Lucy Puryear, M.D., and Lauren Marangell, M.D., both of Baylor College of Medicine in Houston, Texas, and Deborah Sichel, M.D. of the Hestia Institute in Wellesley, Massachusetts, are providing pregnant and postpartum mothers with fish oil supplements. As of this writing, the studies are still in progress, but omega-3 fatty acid proponents are hopeful that such supplements will significantly reduce the depression experienced by new mothers around the world. At this point it is not clear if DHA, EPA, or both will have mood-elevating properties in postpartum depression.

Pregnant women should let their doctors know if they are considering omega-3 fatty acid supplementation. It is important to note that so far, no more than 3.5 grams per day of EPA and DHA combined, have been given to pregnant women in research studies. Nevertheless, Eskimo women traditionally consume an average of 400 grams of seal and fish per day (slightly less than a pound). This translates into 14 grams of EPA and DHA daily.

The New Birth Agenda

It is often the case that bad news leads to worse. The bad news is that modern diets low in omega-3 oils cause some complications of pregnancy, including premature birth. The worse news is that premature babies are at greater risk for damage from omega-3 deficit than babies who go to term, since the fetal brain receives the bulk of its omega-3 complement in the third trimester. Once the premature baby leaves the womb, the supply of omega-3s may become tenuous indeed.

But the solution is at hand: empowered with information, pregnant women can increase their intake of omega-3 oils, especially the long-chain EPA and DHA, circumventing the cascade of problems that start at conception and build for a year or more after birth. The weight of the evidence points overwhelmingly to adding omega-3s. With each new study, the naysayers are finding it increasingly difficult to argue their case. The literature suggests that pregnant women should probably increase the amount of DHA in their diets and possibly take supplements as well. Nevertheless, they should consult their health care professionals regarding the advisability of this. Women who are not breast-feeding and want to give their baby omega-3 fatty acids should check with their child's pediatrician. It is possible to squeeze the contents of a fish oil capsule into infant formula. Babies do not need much, but it is important to realize that DHA and other omega-3s must be balanced with the omega-6, arachidonic acid for optimal growth in a newborn and young child.

It may take a few years, but the formula manufacturers, obstetricians, pediatricians, and nutritionists who set our earliest dietary standards will hopefully soon make omega-3s part of the program for maternal and infant success.

6

Fighting Major Depression with Omega-3 Oils

∽ Can eating more omega-3s really boost our moods? The answer, based on the available scientific and clinical evidence, seems to be a cautious yes. There are four lines of evidence supporting the role of omega-3 essential fatty acids in depression. First, there are compelling population studies linking the eating of large amounts of fish (omega-3 fatty acids) to low rates of major depression. The second line of evidence includes neurochemical studies in animals (looking at brain chemistry). The third line of evidence involves biochemical analyses of omega-3 fatty acids and related compounds in the blood of patients with major depression. Clinical evidence comprises the fourth line. Our double-blind placebo-controlled study of omega-3s in bipolar disorder (manic-depressive illness) revealed strong antidepressant effects in this disorder—one closely related to major depression. The final line of evidence also includes the preliminary uncontrolled clinical studies of prescribing omega-3 fatty acids to depressed patients. Controlled clinical trials of omega-3s in depression are under way at a number of research centers. But before examining the link between omega-3s and depression, it is important to understand just what depression is.

Major depression is not the same thing as sadness or the blues or grief. It is a potentially life-threatening medical illness with clear biological roots and treatments. More precisely, major depression is a biological disorder of the brain, while, at the same time, a product of individual psychology, social circumstances, and spiritual belief.

It is hard to appreciate the profoundly painful nature of major depression if you have never experienced it yourself or empathically connected with someone during an episode. Imagine a mild to moderate major depressive episode, where your mood is predominantly low or depressed for at least two weeks. You have lost interest in and derive little pleasure from your usual activities. It is difficult to motivate yourself to get out of bed and function at your job, or in school, or as a parent. Routine activities of daily life, such as bathing, getting dressed, and fixing meals, are difficult to accomplish because you feel drained of energy. Your appetite and sleep have changed (some people eat and sleep less while others have ravenous appetites and sleep excessively). Basically, life is difficult and painful.

Nearly everyone has experienced elements of major depression. If the symptoms are either too brief in duration or not severe enough to meet the formal diagnostic criteria of major depression, the disorder is termed subclinical depression. Although subclinical depression is not formally considered to be an "illness," it can have an impact on anyone's life. Subclinical depression is being increasingly recognized and treated. People no longer need to be so depressed that they are unable to get out of bed to benefit from help. A person with persistent or episodic periods of subclinical depression may have a treatable disorder known as dysthymia. Dysthymia and subclinical depression are very common and respond to the same treatments recommended for major depression: psychotherapy and antidepressant medications.

In a severe depressive episode, all of the symptoms described above are present, but are amplified. All joy for life has disappeared. Even memories of happier times often cannot be retrieved. The person derives no pleasure from previously enjoyable activities and people. Some people with severe major depression have nearly constant thoughts of suicide or death or tormenting impulses to review their flaws and foibles, and wracking sensations of worthlessness and guilt. Trapped in this despair, they find sleep, appetite, and concentration so dramatically altered they cannot function at work, at school, or in relationships. Their energy is so reduced that even the smallest task requires enormous effort. When they do fall asleep, their dreams may mirror the nightmarish experience of their waking hours and they awake exhausted. Occasionally people can still function in one area—holding it together at work, for instance, and thus masking the severity of the depression.

Most people blame themselves for being depressed. Family and friends may blame the person as well. Patients of mine have reported being yelled at, slapped in the face, and told to just "pull yourself up by your bootstraps." But during major depression, there are no bootstraps. There is no apparent escape. The feelings of helplessness and hopelessness during depressive episodes have been described by a patient of mine as "a black hole." The despair can be limitless and unimaginably painful. In my practice, individuals with major depression often tell me that the psychic pain of their illness pervades every aspect of their existence and is worse than any physical pain they have endured.

This may sound dramatic, but think about the 765,000 suicide attempts and 30,000 suicides in the United States each year. That is 84 suicides a day, or 1 every seventeen minutes, and these are only the official numbers. The actual figures are likely much higher. Many of these individuals see death as the only option—even if they leave behind loved ones, including small children whose lives will be forever scarred by the self-inflicted death of a parent. Looked at another way, various studies have documented that the chance that a person with recurrent episodes of major depression will commit suicide is somewhere between 10 and 15 percent.

Major depression is a biopsychosocial illness, with biological, psychological, social, and even spiritual causes and treatments. It is not the province only of those with especially susceptible genes. Anyone may be hit with trauma and loss that may lead to major depression. Difficult life events such as the death of a loved one, an abusive relationship, a childhood filled with abuse or neglect, poverty, a natural disaster, or a war can cause changes at the psychological, social, spiritual, and biological levels in the human brain. Given how serious major depression can be, anyone who is experiencing a depressed mood that seems beyond what is normal should seek help immediately.

Every person handles psychic stressors differently. Some people weather a loss unscathed, usually after an appropriate period of grief. Others may get swallowed up by the grief and sadness and slip into a major depressive episode. The reaction depends on the interaction of the event or environmental influence itself with the individual's psychological, spiritual, and biological makeup. Some people inherit heavy biological loading from their parents, leaving them vulnerable to depression; for this group, episodes of major depression may strike without warning or provocation. Others are on the opposite side of the biological spectrum; despite seemingly unbearable loss, they do not become persistently or excessively depressed. Most people are somewhere in between with some (unknown) degree of biological vulnerability for depression that could activate under the proper circumstances (see Figure 6–1).

DSM-IV Criteria for Major Depression

After years of debate, there is now general agreement on criteria for diagnosis of major depression, defined by the American Psychiatric Association's *Diagnostic and Statistical Manual of Mental Disorders*, 4th edition (1994), referred to as DSM-IV. Some of the criteria may appear somewhat arbitrary, but some flexibility is built in to the diagnostic system. Because of the complexity and inaccessibility of the brain, most psychiatric disorders have unknown biological causes. So, unlike many medical illnesses, where a precise abnormality in a specific organ system can be identified, psychiatry has few valid biological markers of diagnosis. For this reason, DSM-IV relies on subjective symptoms and objective clinical signs to make a diagnosis. Despite its flaws, the DSM system of diagnosis is highly reliable for many psychiatric disorders. Until advances in neuroscience reveal the biological roots of psychiatric disorders, the DSM will continue to be the gold standard for psychiatric diagnosis in most countries around the world.

According to DSM-IV, you are depressed if you suffer:

1. Depressed mood or loss of interests for most of the day nearly every day for at least two weeks.
2. Four or more of the following symptoms:
   * Reduced energy
   * Altered sleep patterns (usually insomnia, but sometimes too much sleep)
   * Changes in appetite (usually diminished appetite, though sometimes increased appetite)
   * Difficulty in concentrating
   * Low self-esteem in comparison to the usual level of self-esteem
   * Inappropriate guilt and self-blame
   * Psychomotor agitation (pacing or wringing hands) or retardation (lying around or being unable to move without effort)
   * Thoughts of suicide
3. These symptoms must be severe enough to reduce the person's level of functioning—either at work, at home, or at school.
4. These symptoms are not due to another medical disorder such as low thyroid functioning.

Depression Up, Omega-3 Down: Population Studies

Major depression is one of the most common and deadly of the mental illnesses, afflicting millions of Americans each year; one of every six people can expect to suffer major depression at some point during their lifetime. Moreover, it is on the rise and is affecting more of our children, at younger and younger ages, than at any time in human history. An elegant series of research papers from the husband and wife team of Myrna M. Weissman,

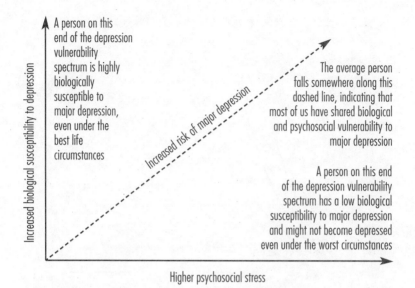

FIGURE 6–1: Spectrum of Psychological and Biological Vulnerability to Major Depression

This figure is a highly schematic model of different vulnerabilities to develop major depression. People above the dotted, diagonal arrow tend to be biologically predisposed to major depression, above and beyond any life events. In contrast, individuals below that line tend to be biologically resistant to becoming depressed; it would take a very large psychosocial stress to induce an episode of major depression. Most people lie somewhere between these two extremes. However, there is currently no way to precisely identify a person's biological vulnerability to becoming depressed.

Ph.D., and the late Gerald L. Klerman, M.D., have provided overwhelming evidence that the worldwide rates of major depression rose in every decade of the twentieth century. What is more, the age of onset for the first episode has gone down in each succeeding decade. This well-documented trend has accelerated since World War II. Those born before 1914, for instance, were about one hundred times less likely to be depressed by the age of forty-five than were those born after 1945 (see Figure 6–2.)

Remarkably, longitudinal studies show that the increased rates of major depression parallel the increase in our diets of seed oils like corn and soy (sources of omega-6) and the corresponding

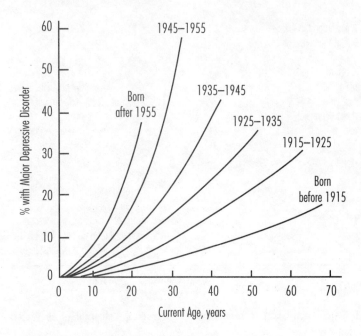

FIGURE 6–2: Increase in Rates of Depression

Researchers have documented an alarming and dramatic rise in the rates of major depression in each subsequent decade of the twentieth century. Perhaps even more worrisome is the steady decrease in the age of onset of major depression in this century. A person born after World War II is at far higher risk of developing major depression at some point during his or her lifetime than a person born earlier in the century. There is likely more than one cause for the increased prevalence of depression. Factors, such as breakdown of the extended family structure, soaring rates of substance abuse, the effects of media and technology, and even toxic pollutants in the environment, may be contributing to the increase in depression. There is now emerging evidence that the steady decline in omega-3 fatty acids in our diet may be a much larger factor in the rise of depression than anyone suspected.

decline in omega-3 fats. Our ancestors, who ate a wide variety of leafy green vegetables, fish, and wild game, consumed omega-3 fatty acids in relatively equal proportion to their biochemical counterparts, the omega-6 fatty acids (such as linoleic acid and arachidonic acid.)

The seed oils, on the other hand, have drastically adverse ratios of omega-6 to omega-3; in corn oil, for instance, omega-6 fatty acids are seventy-five times more plentiful than the omega-3s. This very imbalance could be at the root of the recent disturbing trends in major depression.

The Fish Factor: Eating Fish Is Associated with Lower Rates of Major Depression

The link between depression and lipids has been the special passion of psychiatrist and researcher Joseph R. Hibbeln, M.D., chief of the Outpatient Clinic, Laboratory of Clinical Studies at the National Institute on Alcohol Abuse and Alcoholism and Laboratory of Clinical Studies at the National Institutes of Health in Bethesda, Maryland. Dr. Hibbeln is a leading expert on omega-3 fatty acids and depression. He looked at populations still consuming historically high quantities of omega-3 oils to validate the link.

His defining study, published in 1998 in the prestigious British journal *The Lancet*, compared the annual rates of major depressive illness with levels of fish consumption in a cross section of nations, from France and New Zealand to Japan. To do the work, Hibbeln relied on data from the Klerman and Weissman studies mentioned earlier, which examined rates of depression around the world. Hibbeln also used economic data to estimate how much fish (a rough approximation of omega-3 consumption) was eaten in the different countries where he had data on depression. Of special interest was the finding that among nations, Japan had the lowest apparent rate of depression—a minuscule 0.12 percent while New Zealand, at 6 percent, had the world's highest rate—some fifty times higher than Japan! (Hibbeln's studies were based on annual rates of depression rather than lifetime rates, which are higher.)

Amazingly, he found that differences from country to country could be predicted by how much fish the population ate (see Figure 6–3). In a larger and more recent study (detailed in Chapter 5), Hibbeln found an even stronger association between rates of postpartum depression and lack of fish in the diet in various countries. The less fish a population consumed, the higher the rate of postpartum depression. This finding makes intuitive sense since the pregnant or nursing woman transfers very large quantities of the omega-3 fatty acids to the baby, a requirement for the healthy development of the baby's brain and nervous system. If the mother's diet is inadequate, the transfer of omega-3 fatty acids to her baby may result in maternal omega-3 depletion, which presumably leaves her vulnerable to a range of medical disorders, including depression.

As compelling as these studies are, caution should be exercised in assuming causality. Dr. Hibbeln's data showed an *association* between fish consumption and lower rates of depressive illness. Only careful, controlled intervention studies can prove causality—the cause-and-effect relationship between two factors. For example, in the Asian countries where the Klerman and Weissman rates of major depression were low, there is the possibility of a culturally mediated underreporting of depressive symptoms. Nevertheless, the associations detected in epidemiological studies can be quite compelling. However, an association may be due to causality, coincidence, or some other reason. For instance, fatal car accidents are extremely rare for people who own Volvos. Thus, you may conclude that Volvos protect occupants better than other cars during a crash, *or* that people who buy Volvos are safer drivers. Causality is often assumed (Volvos are safer cars) when only an association (fewer fatalities in Volvos) has been observed. This tendency must be overcome when assessing scientific research. Nonetheless, associations are surely suggestive and especially valuable as guides for researchers looking for causal factors.

Hibbeln was also fascinated by the longstanding observation that major depression and heart disease are linked. Not only are individuals with major depression at greater risk for heart disease in general, but a depressed individual who has a heart attack is also much more likely to die of arrhythmias or blood clots. For decades, researchers have been asking the chicken and the egg question: does depression cause heart disease or does heart disease cause depression? Hibbeln suspected the answer was none of the above.

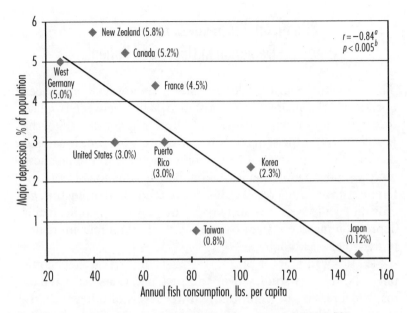

FIGURE 6–3: Fish Consumption and Major Depression Around the World

This graph depicts the surprising association between the amount of fish a country consumes and that nation's rates of major depression. Countries that eat more fish have lower rates of major depression. There may be several possible explanations for this observation, but the most compelling is that the relatively high levels of omega-3 fatty acids in the bodies and brains of the citizens of fish-eating countries protect against depression.

Notes: [a]r = statistical correlation. [b]p = level of statistical significance. Any value <0.05 is considered statistically significant.

Instead, he looked to the fatty acid research for a clue. Enough research data had been published in cardiology to indicate that the severity of heart disease was associated with low levels of omega-3 fatty acids. The psychiatric literature has also recently published studies indicating that the presence and severity of major depression are also associated with low levels of omega-3s. As with depression, heart disease is approximately fifty times more prevalent in nations with low levels of fish consumption as compared to countries at the top of the fish-eating scale. It only makes sense, he notes, to trace both illnesses to the single, shared cause of omega-3 fatty acid deficiency.

Bad Blood: Biochemical Evidence of
Omega-3 Depletion in Depressed Patients

The epidemiological evidence, although powerful, has been open to attack. An association or statistical link between two factors does not prove a cause-and-effect relationship. Do the Japanese truly experience less major depression and, if so, is it due to culture, genetics, or some other factor? Do the Japanese merely report depression less often, perhaps due to cultural differences from the West? Hibbeln contends that even though crowding and stress are constants for the Japanese people, major depression may be kept at bay due to the harmonious influence of the omega-3s.

Skeptics want harder proof, of course, and researchers complied. Numerous studies over the past few years have linked major depression to significantly lower levels of omega-3 fatty acids in the blood:

- Peter B. Adams and his colleagues at the Rockhampton Base Hospital and the Centre for Mental Health Research in Melbourne, Australia, have shown that the severity of depressive symptoms was associated with higher blood levels of omega-6 fatty acids (arachidonic acid) compared to lower blood levels of omega-3 EPA.

- Michael Maes of the University Hospital of Antwerp in Belgium has shown that low levels of omega-3 fatty acids in the blood serum are associated with major depression. Those with major depression, he reported, also had significantly less EPA in the lipoproteins in the blood that carry cholesterol than those with minor depression. This suggests, he adds, that major depression may potentially be related to "an abnormal intake or metabolism" of these essential nutrients.

- Studying fifty patients hospitalized after attempting suicide, Hibbeln found that in the patients without major depression, having high levels of EPA was associated with less severe symptoms of depression on six different rating scales. This study suggests that some patients may reduce the severity of their depressive or suicidal symptoms by taking EPA supplements.

* Malcolm Peet of the University of Sheffield in the United Kingdom has found that the red blood cell membranes of depressed patients are depleted of omega-3 fatty acids, especially the long-chain DHA molecule, critical to functioning of the brain.

These biochemical studies on plasma and red blood cell levels of omega-3 are compelling, but like the epidemiological research, these associations still do not constitute a cause-and-effect relationship between low levels of omega-3 fatty acids and major depression.

Theory of the Blues: Neurochemical Data in Animals and Omega-3 Fatty Acids

The ultimate evidence linking the different omega-3s and depression will emerge through a combination of double-blind, placebo-controlled studies and further exploration of neurochemistry, revealing what brain pathways are altered when the omega-3 fatty acids are absent. It is already known that omega-3 fatty acids are fundamental to the nervous system. DHA and EPA appear to be crucial to the structure and activity of the brain from the earliest days in the womb.

The most widely accepted theory regarding the biology of major depression involves a dysregulation or abnormality of specific brain chemicals, most notably the neurotransmitters serotonin, norepinephrine, and dopamine. Details regarding the presumed brain abnormalities in depression remain unclear. In fact, clues leading to the current theories of major depression come mainly from the serendipitous discovery of effective antidepressants over the years. Working backward, scientists then try to determine which biochemical mechanisms in the brain are influenced by the antidepressant drug. For example, if a new and effective antidepressant affects the neurotransmitter serotonin, then it is reasonable to assume that serotonin must be involved somehow in major depression. A more detailed picture may emerge from animal studies, where analyzing brain chemistry is easier and more direct than it is in humans.

The omega-3 fatty acids are an integral part of the structure and function of the brain. The brain does not function well unless adequate amounts of omega-3 fatty acids circulate in the bloodstream and are incorporated into cell membranes. Omega-3 fatty acids also appear to influence the brain chemicals involved in antidepressant action. For example, French scientists have shown that rats deficient in omega-3 fatty acids had more receptors for the neurotransmitter serotonin and a corresponding decrease in dopamine in the frontal cortex. The direction of the changes in these neurotransmitter systems is consistent with some human models of major depression. Not surprisingly, other scientists have observed that increasing the dietary intake of omega-3 fatty acids boosted the levels of the neurotransmitter dopamine in the frontal cortex of rats. In humans, increased dopamine in the frontal cortex increases drive and motivation, attributes lacking in the depressed person. The box entitled "Omega-3 Fatty Acids and the Depressed Brain" shows some of the current hypotheses regarding the mechanisms of action of DHA, EPA, and ALA relating to mood.

Based on these and other observations, omega-3 oils might be compared to the antidepressant Prozac, the first of several selective serotonin reuptake inhibitor (SSRI) antidepressants introduced in the United States. The initial mechanism of action of drugs like Prozac is to block the neurons' reuptake (the recycling and deactivation of a neurotransmitter) of serotonin, leaving more serotonin available in the synapse between cells to deliver its chemical message from cell to cell throughout the brain. Of course, the biochemistry of major depression is far more complicated than one neurotransmitter, yet based on the relatively simple serotonin theory of depression, the drug Prozac was born. Millions of people around the world have been treated with Prozac and the other new antidepressants. Many of these individuals have obtained substantial relief from their depressive symptoms. In a similar way, the omega-3 depletion theory of depression may yield a new and safer class of antidepressant treatments: fish oil and other sources of omega-3 fatty acids, providing the benefits without negative side effects.

Yet the omega-3s and the EPA-derived eicosanoids are not limited in their action to merely serotonin. They act in many ways, ranging from altering levels of stress hormones, such as cortisol, to actually changing the electrical properties of neurons. One of the most exciting new areas of research is the study of the effects of omega-3 and eicosanoid receptors on the nucleus of cells. This indicates that the omega-3s and the omega-6s are working at the most profound level of cell functioning by directly acting on the nucleus to change gene expression.

Omega-3 Fatty Acids and the Depressed Brain

There are many mechanisms currently thought to be involved in the antidepressant effects of the omega-3s. Each possible mechanism is involved in mood regulation. Our full understanding of omega-3 fatty acid action in depression will require many more studies; however, it is likely that the omega-3s act in several concurrent ways to boost and stabilize mood, possibly with mechanisms of action yet to be discovered.

Potential mechanisms of action of omega-3 fatty acids in depression and bipolar disorder:

- EPA is converted into different eicosanoids, such as prostaglandins, leukotrienes, and thromboxanes. EPA and its eicosanoid derivatives may directly affect mood via specific receptors in the brain.

- EPA competes with arachidonic acid, its omega-6 counterpart, modulating the effect of AA and thus preventing the formation of powerful immune chemicals known as cytokines. Cytokines, in combination with an exaggerated inflammatory response, can depress mood, possibly through abnormal activation of the hypothalamic-pituitary axis, affecting hormones, such as cortisol and thyroid hormone.

- DHA, EPA, and ALA decrease the inflammatory response and mitigate cytokine action, in part, through inhibition of enzymes, such as cycloxygenase (cox-1, cox-2), responsible for inflammation, pain, and possibly mood.

- DHA and EPA alter the process of signal transduction in brain cells in a variety of ways. Signal transduction is the process in which the information from the neurotransmitter-receptor interaction in the synapse is transmitted into the cell, leading to a cascade of biochemical events, ultimately controlling many different aspects of cell activity, including gene expression and neurotransmitter activity.

- EPA, acting in the phospholipid cell membrane's inner leaflet inhibits the action of phosphatidylinositol-specific phospholipase C in humans, reducing the generation of second messenger molecules. In addition, the omega-3s have been recently shown to inhibit two crucial cell-signaling molecules: G-proteins and protein kinase C.

- EPA, DHA, and eicosanoids can directly activate receptors in the nucleus, called peroxisomal proliferater activated receptors (PPARs), leading to changes in gene expression, perhaps affecting mood.

- DHA, EPA, and ALA all affect calcium, sodium, and potassium ion channels, which are crucial for regulating cellular electrical activity, particularly in the heart and brain. This ion current modulation occurs in excitable tissue by omega-3 interaction with binding sites on the proteins comprising the ion channel. This modulation generally results in the cells being less responsive to electrical events and reduces abnormal electrical activity.

- DHA, EPA, and ALA are incorporated into the cell membrane, where they affect the physical structure and fluidity of the membrane. This in turn leads to changes in the function of various cell structures embedded in the membrane, including receptors for neurotransmitters, such as serotonin.

Depression and the Immune Response: The Mind-Body Connection

The fourth line of evidence in the connection of depression to an omega-3 deficiency is the link between mood disorders and the brain's immune and inflammatory pathways. The deficiency of omega-3 fatty acids in our diet places all of us, including our children, at higher risk for developing depression and a range of other medical problems, particularly those involving the immune system. Depression is occurring in children at progressively younger ages. Currently over half a million children are on prescription antidepressants.

Asthma is also on the rise in children, as is rheumatoid arthritis and other immune/inflammatory disorders in adults. How do the increases in these immune system-mediated illnesses possibly relate to the increased rates of depression? The answer may lie in the profound effects that eicosanoids and omega-3s have on immune function. The deficiency of omega-3s, particularly EPA, leaves the body exposed to the dangerous overactivation of the immune system caused by unchecked omega-6 fatty acids. Michael Maes and others have built a convincing body of evidence demonstrating this connection between the immune system, the inflammatory response and depression.

The Inflammatory Process

This fourth line of biological evidence connecting depression to omega-3 depletion demonstrates the necessity for the balance of omega-6 to omega-3 in the body. Omega-6 fatty acids are obtained from seed and vegetable oils that have increased in our diet through the incorporation of these oils by the food industry, at the early recommendations of the American Heart Association and others. Omega-6 arachidonic acid competes with the omega-3 EPA to achieve a balanced immune function in health. Like EPA, arachidonic acid is converted to a series of eicosanoids, including prostaglandins and leukotrienes. AA, EPA, and eicosanoids are also important in the formation of cytokines, powerful immune activators. The Nobel Prize in Medicine was awarded in 1982 to Sune K. Bergstrom, Bengt I. Samuelsson, and Sir John R. Vane, for their discovery in the 1960s of the prostaglandins and their powerful effects in the inflammatory process and the immune response. With the initial focus on the eicosanoids derived from omega-6 fatty acids and arachidonic acid, the relevance of the corresponding and counterbalancing omega-3 EPA eicosanoids was initially overlooked.

Omega-6 and omega-3 essential fatty acids are meant to be in a 1 to 1 ratio, placing the omega-6 AA in balance with the omega-3 EPA. According to William E. M. Landes, Ph.D., at the National Institute of Alcohol Abuse and Alcoholism at NIH, the eicosanoids from arachidonic acid are synthesized in an explosive, fast response and likewise have intense and powerful actions in the body. Eicosanoids derived from the omega-3 EPA are created more slowly and their actions are often moderate in comparison to the omega-6 eicosanoids. The parent AA and EPA and their eicosanoids compete directly with each other for receptor sites, modulating the function of many different systems. Without sufficient EPA, arachidonic acid and its progeny will occupy the eicosanoid receptor sites throughout the body, producing a higher risk of an intense, unchecked inflammatory response. Such an imbalance toward the omega-6 eicosanoids causes white blood cells to release potent immune-activating cytokines, which if chronically or abnormally activated will adversely affect health and mood. The consequence of excessive AA-derived eicosanoids is disproportionate inflammation and abnormally elevated cytokines specific to each organ system in the body. With the current ratio of omega-6 to omega-3 being as much as 10 to 20 to 1, what Americans call health is likely to be a state of constant inflammatory immune activation.

The Macrophage and Depression

Depression may be one result of the dysregulated and complex inflammatory response due to high levels of the omega-6 AA and low levels of the omega-3 EPA. Smith was the first to consider the possibility that an imbalance in omega-6 to omega-3 essential fatty acid ratio might cause depression in his "Macrophage Theory of Depression." The word "macrophage" means "big eater" in Greek, and big eaters they are. A macrophage is a large white blood cell deployed by the immune system to engulf and digest invading bacteria, viruses, damaged cells, and other biological "refuse." The macrophage is also a prodigious chemical factory. When macrophages are working normally, they produce optimal quantities of such healthy molecules as human growth hormone, interferon (a cytokine), and the mood-elevating endorphins, the body's natural morphine. But if aspects of the immune/inflammation system are out of balance, suggests Smith in a journal called Medical Hypotheses, the macrophages may secrete excessive quantities of cytokines and other inflammatory molecules. Excessive production of some of these molecules—particularly interferon and some interleukins—are now known to cause bouts of major depression.

Maes and other scientists at the Clinical Research Center for Mental Health, in Antwerp, Belgium, and the Laboratory of Biological Psychiatry at Case Western Reserve University in Cleveland, Ohio, report that the core of the uncontrolled inflammatory response effect on the brain of people with major depression is the overproduction of specific omega-6 arachidonic acid eicosanoids and their corresponding cytokines. Three cytokines affecting the brain regions mediating mood are interleukin β (IL-1), IL-6, and tumor necrosis factor. Among other actions, these cytokines activate the hypothalamus at the base of the brain, which then stimulates the pituitary and adrenal glands to churn out stress hormones such as cortisol (a corticosteroid). Corticosteroids can cause either depression or mania and also impair immunity. The pro-inflammatory cytokines are also thought to be activated in the presence of various stressors, such as cancer or a heart attack. This may explain the increase in depression observed in certain cancers or after a stroke or heart attack.

The omega-3 essential fatty acids, particularly EPA and its eicosanoids, can suppress both the abnormal inflammatory response and abnormal cytokine production. In our current state of widespread omega-3 deficiency, vulnerable individuals may develop depression to any number of internal or external stressors, possibly through activation of the cytokine response.

In the disease lupus, the abnormal inflammatory response produced, in part, by the overabundance of omega-6 arachidonic acid produces a mixed state of immune suppression and immune activation. Lupus is also associated with depression. In this mixed state, cytokines cause certain central nervous system functions to spin out of control, affecting mood, cognitive functioning, and behavior. When given to normal volunteers or to patients with a variety of medical disorders, the cytokines IL-1 or interferon induce symptoms identical to severe major depression. Patients with diseases associated with macrophage and inflammatory activation, from cancer to cardiovascular disease to neurological disorders, have far higher rates of major depression than the general population.

The activity of the neurotransmitter serotonin, vital to mood regulation, is also dramatically altered by the same cytokines. These cytokines also decrease the serotonin precursor L-tryptophan, circulating in the blood, diminishing the body's ability to rebuild serotonin supplies. These omega-6 eicosanoid and cytokine mediated actions on serotonin could lead to depression.

It is possible that increased dietary EPA could alleviate these symptoms by checking the cytokine output.

Promoting an Anti-inflammatory State

Omega-3 fatty acids challenge the omega-6 fatty acids and promote an anti-inflammatory state. One study revealed one of the mechanisms of this EPA-mediated suppression. Researchers at Brigham and Women's Hospital in Boston gave healthy individuals high doses of EPA and DHA in a study of the activation of leukotrienes, an inflammatory eicosanoid molecule. They demonstrated for the first time that EPA alone, not DHA, inhibited the leukotriene activation pathway by suppressing the cell's signaling processes.

Prior to this study the small amount of EPA in the cell membrane had not been recognized as having an active function other than structural support. This study showed that EPA from the membrane was released to actively suppress the inflammatory responses. Circulating EPA also inhibited the inflammatory response. Dietary supplementation of EPA increased EPA in cells, demonstrating that omega-3 dietary supplementation can profoundly affect immune function.

Although speculative, the inflammatory theory of depression may unify a host of observations that were previously unexplained. It is also consistent with the theory that the soaring rates of major depression in this century are mediated by the rising ratios in our diets of omega-6 fatty acids relative to omega-3s. Based on this theory, it seems prudent for a health-care provider treating a patient with major depression to be suspicious of underlying illnesses possibly associated with inflammatory activation. It also should spur us on to test predictions that omega-3 oils can successfully prevent and/or treat not only depressive disorders, but also other illnesses possibly associated with immune dysregulation.

The Real *Feel-Good Food:*
Salmon Steak or Cookie Dough? *Cholesterol and Mood*

For those of a certain mind-set, there is nothing like a tub of Häagen-Dazs or a box of Mallomars to drive depression away. The notion of cholesterol as a low-tech Prozac has its proponents, and research has even linked low-cholesterol diets to increased rates of depression and suicide. As an important part of brain cell membranes, it was held, cholesterol deficit could throw the brain off balance and alter the function of serotonin, one of the neurotransmitters central to the disease.

To those who thought about it, it didn't make sense. If low cholesterol raised the risk of depression while reducing the risk of heart disease, then high rates of depression and low rates of heart disease should be paired. In fact, the opposite is true. Depression and heart disease coexist, rising and falling in tandem in study after study and in countries around the world. The recent publication of a Finnish study unable to link cholesterol and depression called the cholesterol theory of brain balance into doubt. If a low cholesterol diet did, in fact, cause depression, the proof was tenuous and the reason unclear.

Now Joseph Hibbeln of the National Institute of Alcohol Abuse and Alcoholism says the mystery may have been solved; a misinterpretation of the data, not any hidden benefits of cholesterol is at the root. One study that showed no link between reduced cholesterol and depression lowered dietary cholesterol by adding fish, enriching the brain with EPA and DHA. Another study linked a low-cholesterol diet to aggression, but did so by increasing the ratio of omega-6 to omega-3 fatty acids almost fivefold. A third study avoided these pitfalls by lowering cholesterol with drugs. But Hibbeln notes that some cholesterol-lowering drugs "bind fats and interfere with fat absorption in the gut. They may interfere with the absorption of essential fatty acids as well as absorption of cholesterol."

> The bottom line is this: cholesterol in any quantity will not cure the blues. If you want a boost, you may just need omega-3s.

The Fish Cure:
The Early Clinical Experience of Lifting Depression with Omega-3 Fatty Acids

Despite the four lines of compelling evidence supporting the omega-3 depletion hypothesis of major depression presented earlier in this chapter, science requires the standard of proof, which is the completion of double-blind, placebo-controlled trials on omega-3 fats in depression, confirming the preliminary studies.

A number of centers in the United States and the United Kingdom are now examining the antidepressant effects of the different omega-3 fatty acids in patients with major depression. However, until the double-blind, placebo-controlled data are available, "open label" clinical data are useful. Open label is the phase of clinical treatment research prior to the controlled trials, when both the doctor and the patient know they are receiving the medication under study.

Open-label studies have the disadvantage of being influenced by the placebo effect or bias, including a conscious or unconscious fudging of the results. Indeed, results might be exaggerated by patients who desperately want to feel better or just please the doctor. They might be stretched, consciously or unconsciously, by researchers who want their "discovery" to work. Even the most trustworthy physicians and honest patients can be influenced on the unconscious level, and such unwitting bias can taint the results.

Despite these shortcomings, open-label studies are the necessary precursors to very expensive and technically difficult placebo-controlled studies. Open-label studies are cheap and fast, and they happen to be the backdrop for almost all exciting medical discoveries. Rigorously controlled, multimillion-dollar studies are not generally the source of discovery, though they are crucial for verification of the results.

The first psychiatrist to publish his open-label experience with an omega-3 fatty acid in neuropsychiatric disorders was Donald O. Rudin, M.D., from Eastern Pennsylvania Psychiatric Institute in Philadelphia. Dr. Rudin's 1981 paper describes giving flaxseed oil (sometimes called linseed oil, a source of ALA, the short-chain omega-3) in high doses to twelve patients with a variety of physical and mental symptoms. Five patients in this series were diagnosed with schizophrenia, four with agoraphobia, and three with bipolar disorder. The three individuals with bipolar disorder each developed hypomania, mania, or increased mood cycling (rapid shifts of mood) when receiving very large doses of flaxseed oil, suggesting possible antidepressant-like or destabilizing effects of ALA. The dosage ranged up to 120 cc per day of flaxseed oil, or more than 50 grams of ALA per day! The results of Dr. Rudin's uncontrolled study were difficult to interpret, partly because his dosage of ALA (flaxseed oil) was five to ten times higher than the dosage of omega-3 (fish oil) used in our bipolar study. Furthermore, ALA may have different effects in the body and the brain than either EPA or DHA. Nonetheless, Dr. Rudin's pioneering work is important; he was one of the first physicians to recognize the possibility that an omega-3 deficiency could be a widespread cause of medical and neuropsychiatric disorders.

Given the extreme safety of the omega-3s and the positive results in our study of bipolar disorder, showing that omega-3 fatty acids are helpful for depression, I began prescribing them in open-label fashion for sixteen patients with treatment-resistant major depression. We term these patients "treatment-resistant," because they had not responded to numerous past trials on standard antidepressant medication. I added a daily dosage of omega-3 fatty acids (either fish oil or flaxseed oil) to their ongoing antidepressant medication.

We found the results encouraging. Five of sixteen responded at least partially, and four of those experienced marked improvement when omega-3 was added to their ongoing antidepressant treatment. While five of sixteen (22 percent) may not seem impressive, it is important to realize these were treatment-resistant cases, where response rates are usually quite low, often well below 10 percent.

The patients who responded to the omega-3 oils were themselves quite surprised. However, if you think about it, perhaps the very treatment-resistant cases are among those who should respond to omega-3s. This may be because without omega-3 fatty acids, the brain cannot function normally, so even the most powerful antidepressant will be unable to improve mood. For these resistant patients, the brain might be compared to a race car—with powerful fuel as the metaphor for that powerful antidepressant and spark plugs as the metaphor for the omega-3s. Without spark plugs, even the best fuel will be useless.

Wanted: Double-Blind Proof

A definitive statement cannot be made about the antidepressant effects of the different omega-3 fatty acids until the results of ongoing, well-controlled clinical trials are in. Nonetheless, looking at all the omega-3 data, compelling and independent lines of evidence support a role for these oils in the origin, physiology, and pharmacology of major depression. The independent lines of evidence, from epidemiology and basic neurochemistry to open-label data and direct measurement of omega-3 deficiency in the blood, all point to a crucial role for the omega-3 fatty acids in the regulation of mood. Taken together, they may herald a new era in the understanding, prevention, and treatment of depression.

The Mood-Boosting Diet

Understanding that definite proof is not yet in, if you want to use diet to improve your mood you might start by adjusting your diet to include foods high in omega-3 fatty acids, especially the long-chain molecules, eicosapentanoic acid (EPA) and possibly docosahexanoic acid (DHA). The Omega-3 Renewal Program guides you step by step in how to incorporate a mood-enhancing diet into your life. An excellent way to start is simply to begin eating more fish. Fatty species, such as salmon, have more EPA and DHA than lean fish. Many experts suggest people eat two to three fish meals a week to reduce cardiac risk. The amount of omega-3 required in food or supplement form to elevate mood remains unknown, but is possibly higher than that needed in the periphery.

If you want to add supplements, again the Omega-3 Renewal Plan will provide information for you. Self-treatment of serious depression is dangerous. Moreover, the omega-3 fatty acids are powerful molecules, and one should respect the alterations in mood that can accompany a large dietary change. This book is intended to provide information; it is not meant to replace careful evaluation or treatment by a physician. Find a doctor or health-care professional who can work with you to adjust the food in your diet, to determine the proper dosage of omega-3 supplements and/or conventional medications, if indicated. Bring the book in to your doctor if you think it will be useful. Under no circumstance should you stop prescription medication unless you and your clinician agree on this course. The simplest course is to add omega-3 fatty acids to whatever ongoing treatment you are receiving.

7

Omega-3 and Bipolar Disorder

୬ In May 1999, my colleagues and I published the first scientifically rigorous clinical trial of omega-3 fatty acids in psychiatry. In this four-month study, we observed that omega-3 fatty acids from fish oil improved and stabilized mood in a group of thirty patients with bipolar disorder, when compared to a matched group of bipolar patients who received a placebo. Finding safer and more effective treatments for my patients and the millions of other people with the fascinating and potentially deadly illness known as bipolar disorder (or manic-depressive illness) was the inspiration for the discovery.

What Is Bipolar Disorder?

Bipolar disorder, also known as manic-depressive illness, is a common and sometimes lethal medical condition. Patients with bipolar disorder suffer from mania, a dangerous elevation of mood into euphoria and irritability, combined with high energy, impulsive and sometimes dangerous behaviors, and a constellation of other symptoms. These patients also often suffer from re-

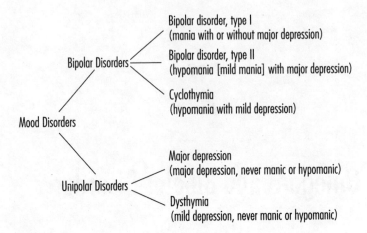

FIGURE 7–1: Classification and Diagnostic Criteria of Mood Disorders

current bouts of major depression of the sort described in the previous chapter.

DSM-IV Criteria for Bipolar Disorder
I. Manic Episode

A. A distinct period of abnormally and persistently elevated, expansive, or irritable mood, lasting at least one week (or any duration if hospitalization is necessary).
B. During the period of mood disturbance, three (or more) of the following symptoms have persisted (four if the mood is only irritable) and have been present to a significant degree:
　1. inflated self-esteem or grandiosity
　2. decreased need for sleep (e.g., feels rested after only three hours of sleep)
　3. more talkative than usual or pressure to keep talking
　4. flight of ideas or subjective experience that thoughts are racing

5. distractibility (i.e., attention too easily drawn to unimportant or irrelevant external stimuli)
6. increase in goal-directed activity (either socially, at work or school, or sexually) or psychomotor agitation
7. excessive involvement in pleasurable activities that have a high potential for painful consequences (e.g., engaging in unrestrained buying sprees, sexual indiscretions, or foolish business investments)

C. The symptoms do not meet criteria for a mixed episode.

D. The mood disturbance is sufficiently severe to cause marked impairment in occupational functioning or in usual social activities or relationships with others, or to necessitate hospitalization to prevent harm to self or others, or there are psychotic features.

E. The symptoms are not due to the direct physiological effects of a substance (e.g., a drug of abuse, a medication, or other treatment) or a general medical condition (e.g., hyperthyroidism).

Note: Manic-like episodes that are clearly caused by somatic antidepressant treatment (e.g., medication, electroconvulsive therapy, light therapy) should not count toward a diagnosis of bipolar I disorder.

II. Hypomanic Episode

A. A distinct period of persistently elevated, expansive, or irritable mood, lasting at least four days that is clearly different from the usual nondepressed mood.

B. During the period of mood disturbance, three (or more) of the following symptoms have persisted (four if the mood is only irritable) and have been present to a significant degree:
1. inflated self-esteem or grandiosity
2. decreased need for sleep (e.g., feels rested after only three hours of sleep)

    3. more talkative than usual or pressure to keep talking

    4. flight of ideas or subjective experience that thoughts are racing

    5. distractibility (i.e., attention too easily drawn to unimportant or irrelevant external stimuli)

    6. increase in goal-directed activity (either socially, at work or school, or sexually) or psychomotor agitation

    7. excessive involvement in pleasurable activities that have a high potential for painful consequences (e.g., engaging in unrestrained buying sprees, sexual indiscretions, or foolish business investments)

C. The episode is associated with an unequivocal change in functioning that is uncharacteristic of the person when not symptomatic.

D. The disturbance in mood and the change in functioning are observable by others.

E. The episode is not severe enough to cause marked impairment in social or occupational functioning or to necessitate hospitalization, and there are no psychotic features.

F. The symptoms are not due to the direct physiological effects of a substance (e.g., a drug of abuse, a medication, or other treatment) or a general medical condition (e.g., hyperthyroidism).

Note: Hypomanic-like episodes that are clearly caused by somatic antidepressant treatment (e.g., medication, electroconvulsive therapy, light therapy) should not count toward a diagnosis of bipolar II disorder.

III. Mixed Episode

A. The criteria are met both for a manic episode and for a major depressive episode (see Chapter 6) (except for duration) nearly every day during at least a one-week period.

B. The mood disturbance is sufficiently severe to cause marked impairment in occupational functioning or in usual social activities or relationships with others, or to necessitate hospitalization to prevent harm to self or others, or there are psychotic features.

C. The symptoms are not due to the direct physiological effects of a substance (e.g., a drug of abuse, a medication, or other treatment) or a general medical condition (e.g., hyperthyroidism).

Note: Mixed episodes that are clearly caused by somatic antidepressant treatment (e.g., medication, electroconvulsive therapy, light therapy) should not count toward a diagnosis of bipolar I disorder.

In the full-blown disorder, periods of suicidal depression may alternate with episodes of mania, including euphoria, irritability, increased energy, decreased need for sleep, and racing thoughts accompanied by impulsive behaviors and grandiose ideas. Symptoms associated with anxiety disorders and even schizophrenia, including hallucinations and delusions, may occur during different phases of the illness. In short, bipolar disorder is a serious, disabling, and sometimes life-threatening brain illness that can include a variety of psychiatric symptoms.

Current Treatments for Bipolar Disorder

The long-term treatment of patients with bipolar disorder relies on the so-called mood stabilizers, such as lithium and valproate. These often produce dramatically good results long term and have doubtless saved thousands of lives. However, in certain patients, serious side effects, the continuation of psychiatric symptoms despite the drugs, and refusal to take their medications were frequent results. This disappointing outcome of the medication treatment is frequently encountered in teaching hospitals like McLean and Brigham and Women's, where many of the patients have severe or treatment-resistant conditions.

Who could blame these people, and those who treat them medically, for being disappointed? As pointed out earlier, lithium has several disadvantages. Many patients who use it experience troublesome weight gain as well as tremors, excessive urination, drowsiness, and acne. A small percentage of its users are likely to develop thyroid and kidney problems. To many of the gifted people who are among its users, its most serious disadvantage is the decrease it brings about in creative energy. Lithium may keep manias within check, but it also flattens emotions. Moreover, many patients require combinations of several mood stabilizers simultaneously to control recurrent manias or depressions, and such combinations increase the risk of drug interactions and harmful side effects.

The search for a cure for bipolar disorder is as old as psychiatry, but it was not until 1949 that a series of accidents ushered in the first real pharmacological hope. Back then, John Cade, a thirty-seven-year-old psychiatrist and superintendent of the Repatriation Mental Hospital in Bundoora, Australia, speculated that mania was caused by a toxic substance manufactured in the body. To find it, he collected urine from his manic patients and, working in the hospital's abandoned pantry, injected it into the bellies of guinea pigs. When the guinea pigs all died, Cade decided to dilute the urine to reduce the toxic uric acid content, and try again. Reckoning (mistakenly) that adding the element lithium would aid in dissolving the uric acid, he tested lithium itself on the guinea pigs. Guinea pigs are known for their dramatic startle reaction when placed on their backs, but Cade's lithium-treated guinea pigs were remarkably placid.

Acting on a hunch, Cade decided to try lithium therapy on his patients, including ten with mania, six with schizophrenia, and three diagnosed with psychotic depression. The lithium did nothing for the depressed patients, but it calmed the schizophrenic patients—and its impact on those with mania was dramatic. All ten showed significant improvement, and five were able to leave the hospital pronounced well.

Of course, nothing is ever that simple. Even administered correctly, lithium's side effects can be intolerable; and if the dosage is too high, lithium can be lethal. That point was hardly missed by critics in 1949. In that year, while Cade's study, published in a small medical journal from Australia, went virtually unnoticed, the *Journal of the American Medical Association* reported that two patients with heart failure had died after receiving lithium as a salt substitute. Lithium had political problems as well: a natural salt that could not be protected by patent, lithium held little attraction for the profit-driven pharmaceutical industry so crucial to drug development. It would take twenty years for psychiatrists to standardize treatment with lithium and for the FDA to approve it for use with bipolar disorder in the United States, and yet another twenty years for only the second mood stabilizer, Depakote (valproate), to become approved for use in the United States. Appendix A contains a complete description of currently used mood stabilizers.

The Search for a Better Mood Stabilizer

A rational first step in improving on the current treatments for bipolar disorder (lithium, valproate, and the other so-called mood stabilizers) was understanding just how they worked in the brain. But the vast quantity of data regarding the neurochemical effects of the various mood stabilizers made it difficult to pin the mechanism down. In fact, we had the rare situation of information overload: each mood stabilizer had so many chemical actions that it was not always clear which were key in treating bipolar disorder. I reasoned that we could find the answer in the vast body of material already in the medical literature and public domain. By comparing all the mood-stabilizing drugs on the basis of their known biochemical actions in the brain and body, it might be possible to find one or more common biochemical mechanisms. If one biochemical action was shared by the mood-stabilizing drugs (which are chemically unrelated to one another), it would indicate that this biochemical action was critically important. In fact, this shared biochemical action of the mood stabilizers would likely be related to whatever neurochemical abnormality was present in bipolar disorder.

I began the search in earnest in 1993, when I took the job as Director of Psychopharmacology at Brigham and Women's Hospital in Boston. Working with a colleague of mine, Dr. W. Emanuel Severus, visiting from Germany's Free University of Berlin, we used the medical database Medline to pull up research papers on several of the more well-known mood stabilizers: lithium, valproate, carbamazepine, and verapamil. We also looked at electroconvulsive therapy (ECT or "shock" therapy), because, although ECT is not a pharmaceutical therapy, it was often effective in stabilizing mood as well. We combed through hundreds of papers on the biochemical actions of the mood stabilizers in the brain and elsewhere in the body in humans as well as in animals. We then constructed a comprehensive chart, with mood stabilizers on one axis and the biochemical actions on the other. Viewing our findings, it seemed clear that the core data were already available—if only we could interpret the information in light of bipolar disorder and the brain.

On the most basic level, our search of the literature confirmed that most mood stabilizers operate largely in the membranes and inside the cell, in contrast to most psychiatric drugs, which act on receptors (the molecule on the outside membrane of the cell to which the neurotransmitter binds) and other processes in the synapse (the space between one nerve cell and the next). The mood stabilizers inhibited a range of chemical reactions, all involved in some way in completing the processes that the neurotransmitters (the brain's chemical messengers) and receptors had begun.

Particularly notable, the mood stabilizers inhibited G-proteins and phospholipases, which are proteins and enzymes that transform phospholipids in the membrane into signaling molecules. These specialized molecules sit on the inside of the cell membrane on the "receiving" neuron and are intended to amplify the original neurotransmitter signal. When a neurotransmitter binds to a receptor, the receptor sets in motion within the cell a series of chemical processes known as signal transduction, amplifying the original signal and ultimately altering the activity of the cell. Different mood stabilizers inhibited different aspects of the biochemical cascade of signal transduction. Inhibiting signal transduction in bipolar disorder would be analagous to building a dam across a raging river, quieting the downstream waters. Presumably the mood stabilizer inhibition of signal transduction in a crucial region of the brain would normalize whatever biochemical process has gone awry in bipolar disorder.

The brain's neurons are like a network of telephone wires carrying signals along their length. Some neurons are extremely long, connecting distant regions, and others are short, reaching out to communicate with many other nerve cells in their immediate vicinity. Nerve cells do not communicate with each other through direct contact. Instead, there's a microscopic gap, the synapse, between the end of one cell and the beginning of another (see figure 7-2). In order for two nerve cells to communicate, neurotransmitters produced by the first cell must cross the synapse and attach to receptor molecules on the membrane of the second cell. That membrane is called the postsynaptic membrane. When certain neurotransmitters bind to receptors in sufficient strength, they set in motion a series of reactions that alter mood and activity in the brain. Transduction is the process by which the chemical signal at the receptor crosses the cell membrane, setting in motion a series of complex biochemical and electrical reactions in the second cell (see figure 7-3).

Looking for Answers: The Promise of Omega-3 Fatty Acids

The basic research showing that individual mood stabilizers inhibit signal transduction was carried out by numerous psychiatric and neuroscience investigators. This apparent common mechanism—the inhibition of signal transduction—was the lead we were searching for in our quest to find new mood-stabilizing compounds for our patients with bipolar disorder. We again searched the medical database Medline, this time looking for chemical compounds that inhibit signal transduction but had

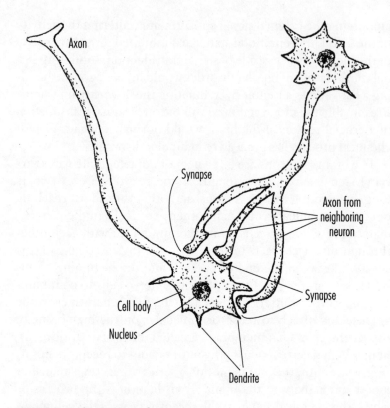

FIGURE 7–2: The Anatomy of a Neuron

The basic units of the brain are the nerve cells, or neurons. Each neuron has four parts:

1. The cell body, including the cell nucleus and its DNA. The cell body manufactures the cell's proteins and many of the substances it needs to function.
2. The axon—the long, tubular extension that carries nerve impulses away from the cell.
3. The dendrites—shorter structures positioned along the cell body. Cell receptors, embedded in the dendrites, receive messages from neurotransmitters crossing the synapse.
4. The synapse—the space between one nerve cell and the next.

never been tested in bipolar disorder. A single group of substances—the omega-3 fatty acids from fish oil—surprisingly emerged as the best candidate to study. The omega-3s had never been formally tested in human neuropsychiatric disorders, but they seemed to have enormous potential based on animal and

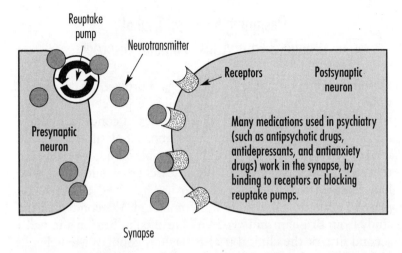

FIGURE 7–3: Neurotransmitter Signal Transmission Between Two Brain Cells

human research. Whether incorporated into cell membranes or circulating in the blood, the omega-3 fatty acids shared biochemical actions with the mood stabilizers in a number of crucial ways and also had independent biochemical actions that could potentially affect mood. As we read more and more data on the omega-3 fatty acids, the possibility that these simple compounds could help our patients became more and more likely.

All in all, an incredible fact seems to have fallen through the cracks of neuroscience and psychiatry: all cell membranes are made of fat, and the omega-3 fatty acids, though depleted in many of us, are supposed to be the most abundant of the essential lipids in the membranes of the brain.

We had no hard evidence that omega-3 fatty acids would be useful in bipolar disorder, but we were optimistic. The next step was to perform a clinical trial to test our ideas.

Designing a Clinical Trial of
Omega-3 Fatty Acids in Bipolar Disorder

Despite no direct funding for an omega-3 project, we designed a nine-month controlled study. It would be placebo-controlled, with half of the patients receiving capsules of concentrated fish oil and the other half receiving a placebo, a look-alike inert pill, made from olive oil. And it would be double-blind, which meant that neither the patients nor the researchers would know who had received the fish oil and who had received the olive oil placebo until after the study was completed. We conducted the study from Brigham and Women's Hospital in Boston and had a second site for the clinical trial at Baylor School of Medicine in Houston, Texas, led by Dr. Lauren B. Marangell, Chief of Psychopharmacology at Baylor.

Our notion of testing fish oil was met with quite a bit of skepticism and friendly teasing from colleagues. However, once we explained the rationale behind using the omega-3 fatty acids as mood stabilizers based on their biochemical actions, people generally thought the idea was interesting. We convinced the National Institutes of Health (NIH) to provide us with a concentrated version of omega-3 fatty acids used in its fish oil initiative for heart disease and other disorders. The fish oil that NIH provided to us was in the form of 1,000-milligram capsules of fish oil, formulated to have a concentration of 70 percent omega-3 fatty acids—much higher than the concentration of typical commercial fish oil available at the time. NIH worked with the National Marine Fisheries in South Carolina to produce this very high-quality oil.

Finally we recruited our test subjects: thirty individuals with bipolar disorder. We chose patients who were at high risk of relapse (including patients with "rapid cycling," characterized by frequent episodes of mania and depression) to maximize our chances of seeing an effect of the omega-3 fatty acids during the study. Had we chosen patients whose bipolar illness was stable, even a placebo would seem to be effective during the relatively short duration of the study. Hence, we selected patients with unstable and difficult-to-treat bipolar disorder.

We had no trouble finding volunteers because existing treatments are often inadequate, the side effects of the omega-3s are relatively few, and omega-3 fatty acids are attractive because they are "natural." Due to the severity of their bipolar disorder, most of those who came to us were on at least one mood stabilizer already, and many were receiving two or more. However, eight subjects were not on any medication at all when they were recruited for the study, either because they objected to drugs or because the conventional treatments produced intolerable side effects or had failed to help.

The study proceeded well. When a large group of subjects had reached the four-month mark, we performed a preplanned preliminary analysis of the data. To our amazement, we found a significant discrepancy between the omega-3 fatty acid group and the placebo control group. Many of the participants receiving omega-3 fatty acid supplements had experienced dramatic recoveries; those receiving placebos were languishing—either failing to recover or relapsing into disease. At about the same time, NIH informed us that the fish oil was no longer going to be manufactured, and we would probably have to cut the study short of the originally planned nine months. Because of the positive results, we decided to end the study when thirty subjects had reached the four-month point. With the group of patients receiving the omega-3 fatty acids doing so much better, it seemed unethical to withhold omega-3 fatty acids from the placebo group suffering from this disabling and potentially lethal disease. Instead, we offered omega-3 fatty acids to all our volunteers—and set out to report the results to the world.

Perhaps because our findings were so unexpected and dramatic, acceptance proved challenging. Presenting our results at a neuroscience research meeting in 1997 (the American College of Neuropsychopharmacology), we were greeted with a mixture of excitement, encouragement, and teasing, including the requisite fish oil jokes. However, the *Archives of General Psychiatry*, one of the leading journals in the field, published our paper.

Clinical Implications

In my practice, the omega-3 fatty acids have emerged as a powerful new intervention for patients with bipolar disease. In the aftermath of our study, NIH gave us their remaining fish oil supplies, and we distributed them to our patients. Virtually all of the study participants elected to stay on or switch to fish oil. To date, I have used, or consulted on the use of, fish oil in the treatment of hundreds of patients, usually using it in addition to lithium, valproate, and other mood stabilizers. For those with milder forms of the disorder, and rarely in more severe cases, I have used the omega-3 fatty acids alone.

I must emphasize that our study represents only one step in the path of omega-3 research in psychiatry. Our results must be independently confirmed before we can definitively conclude that omega-3 fatty acids are beneficial in mood disorders. Nonetheless I have seen striking results in many of the patients I see in my practice. In addition, I receive daily E-mails from around the world reporting "miraculous" responses to fish oil. One E-mail from a patient with bipolar disorder read, "The omega-3 fatty acids probably saved my life," and another, "This disorder comes with a host of unquantifiable gifts, from seeing colors to hearing music with a clarity and intensity that the average person will never experience. It also comes with a terrible price that, because of the omega-3 fatty acids, many of us may not have to continue paying." Another woman has been in frequent contact with me regarding how well her daughter has done since receiving the omega-3 fatty acids. In one of her E-mails, she states, "It has been seven days with no antidepressant. I never believed this could be possible—it is definitely a record for my daughter. She has not been off antidepressants for that many days in six years, in fact, going off for one day before fish oil led to immediate suicidal ideation with her screaming for me to kill her . . . For the first time in her entire life she is relaxed and her memory and cognitive abilities have returned—I cannot tell you how fortunate we feel."

There appears to be little reason to withhold omega-3 fatty acids from most patients with bipolar disorder. Physicians must always weigh the risks and benefits of any regimen. If benefit outweighs risk, they usually opt to go forward. With omega-3 fatty acids, the risks are low, and the benefits can be striking.

Again, it must be emphasized that anyone who substantially increases omega-3s in their diet, with either fish, flaxseed, or supplements, should work closely under the supervision of a healthcare professional.

8

The Omega-3 Response
to Stress and Violence

෪ There is some thought-provoking evidence linking omega-3 fatty acid deficit to stress-related anger, aggression, hostility, and violence in animals and humans alike. Like other areas of omega-3 research, the evidence is suggestive but not definitive and has to be viewed with caution.

Omega-3 Deficit and the Origins of Stress

Appropriate levels of stress in response to danger, work, or illness are essential for our survival. Biologists studying the science of life define stress as the internal response of an organism to a changing environment.

Like the alert of pain after an injury, an appropriate stress response is the key to adaptation and flexibility. A mouse not stressed enough to run from a cat will become an afternoon snack. The stress that propels humans to action has enabled us to prevail: to hunt buffalo, safeguard our children, settle habitats, and explore first our planet and then the universe beyond. Without a normal stress response, including the impulse for fight or flight, an organism might not survive. In the Darwinian struggle for survival of the fittest, a healthy stress response is key.

But too much stress can be destructive, leading to illness or depression on the one hand or hostile anger or violent aggression on the other. In the Darwinian sense, too much aggression is just as deadly as too little. A species with members who too frequently kill their peers is likely to drop from the evolutionary charts in a geologic blink. Just as an outsized immune response can spiral into autoimmune disease, so too an outsized stress response can sometimes spiral into rage and violence.

Some recent research shows a possible link between the shortage of omega-3 fatty acids and anger, hostility, and stress. To make the association, Dr. Tomohito Hamazaki of Toyama University in Japan worked not with violent criminals but with normal students under stress. In a series of experiments, Hamazaki set out to see whether fish oil supplements would engender a greater sense of calm prior to exams.

In one study, Hamazaki provided medical students with capsules containing from 1.5 grams to 1.8 grams of the long-chain omega-3, DHA, or a soybean oil placebo for three months prior to the university's exam period. He measured hostility at the start of the experiment and again three months later, immediately prior to exams. To assess hostility, he presented potentially emotionally charged cartoon illustrations of various human interactions with empty bubbles for each person. The students were asked to write dialogue in the bubbles. There was a much higher rate of hostile and aggressive dialogue in the nineteen medical students who received the placebo during the high-stress period as compared to the twenty-two medical students receiving the fish oil supplements. The ratings of the students' hostilities jumped 58 percent in the placebo group but did not change at all in the omega-3 group.

As a further control, Hamazaki studied forty-six normal students to see whether DHA might reduce hostility even when major stressors like exams do not come into play. Here he found that omega-3 fatty acid supplements had no discernible impact on hostility under more ordinary circumstances, leading him to conclude that "DHA controls hostility at times of mental stress. If there is no stressor, hostility levels are stable."

Particularly relevant for those in the West is the fact that prior to working with Hamazaki, the Japanese students averaged about 220 milligrams of DHA a day—about 25 percent of the amount consumed by the greater Japanese population. Americans consume much less, most receiving some 40 milligrams or 50 milligrams of DHA through their diet each day. During the period of the study, students were supplemented with 1.5 additional grams of DHA—that is, 1,500 milligrams, or about seven times more than without the supplements and about thirty times more than consumed by the average American.

Hamazaki has also been able to show the relationship between DHA and stress in mice. In one of his rodent studies, mice were fed a DHA-deficient or a DHA-enriched diet for four weeks. During that time, researchers measured a factor called rearing frequency, a phenomenon in which mice under stress stand up on their hind legs. Rearing frequency was far higher in the DHA-deficient group, possibly indicating greater levels of perceived stress, than in the group with a DHA-rich menu.

Although scientists are cautious about extrapolating from rodent experiments to humans, the mouse model is important; it is currently impossible to chart the direct impact that omega-3 fatty acids have on the living human brain, but invasive measurements can be taken with rodents. In one study, rats fed DHA and EPA together had 40 percent more dopamine in their frontal lobes than did a group of controls. Consistent with this finding, the supplemented animals exhibited significantly reduced movement, suggestive of the possibility that omega-3s might reduce the impulsivity and hyperactivity associated with attention deficit–hyperactivity disorder in humans as well.

Pushing the Violence Envelope

Also interesting is the evidence of a possible link between omega-3 deficiency and habitually violent crime. As far back as 1986, forensic psychiatrist Matti Virkkunen has measured lipid levels in habitually violent and impulsive prison inmates. He did not measure omega-3s but rather a variety of lipids from the omega-6 category. The observation that omega-6 fatty acid levels were high might suggest that omega-3 levels were low.

Bolstering these findings are studies linking acute alcohol intoxication, violence, and suicide. According to Joseph R. Hibbeln of the National Institute on Alcohol Abuse and Alcoholism, alcohol-related violence has sparked increasing concern. Recent studies, for instance, have found evidence of a genetic link between alcoholism and violence, especially in males who experience their first bout of alcoholism before age twenty. "An onset of alcohol dependence before a person's twentieth birthday doubles their likelihood of incarceration for criminal violence," according to Hibbeln, "and quadruples their likelihood of attempted suicide."

The connection between early onset alcoholism and violence, Hibbeln contends, can be traced to irregularities in serotonin, a chemical in the brain that may be at the root of both. Scientists cannot yet directly measure serotonin in the human brain, but they can do the next best thing by tracking fluid drawn from the spinal canal (cerebrospinal fluid).

In numerous studies, scientists on the trail of violence and early onset alcoholism have documented low concentrations of cerebrospinal fluid 5-hydroxyindoleacetic acid (5-HIAA), a biochemical that reflects serotonin activity in the brain. Low concentrations of 5-HIAA have long been reported in early onset alcoholics, impulsive homicidal offenders, and impulsive fire setters. Healthy volunteers with high hostility scores on standard tests also have low 5-HIAA levels. And the 5-HIAA deficit is a powerful predictor of aggression and social incompetence even for nonhuman primates.

Based on research by Hamazaki and others, Hibbeln suspected that 5-HIAA—and, by association, turnover of serotonin in the brain—would be sensitive to the absence or presence of omega-3 fatty acids in the diet. But reviewing the studies to date, he discovered a perplexing fact: people with higher levels of DHA in the blood also had lower levels of the spinal fluid 5-HIAA. The findings were, on their face, the opposite of what he had come to expect. If omega-3 deficiency was to lead to violence, then higher levels of omega-3 should produce normal (not lower) levels of the "violence" marker, 5-HIAA.

Nonetheless, in a recent, carefully controlled study of the phenomenon, Hibbeln confirmed these seemingly contradictory results. As expected, a group of violent and impulsive study participants (half with a history of alcoholism) had lower levels of the serotonin marker 5-HIAA than a group of nonviolent controls but had higher levels of DHA.

The apparent contradiction, Hibbeln suggests, has a reasonable explanation. Researchers studying violent criminals have already documented a defect in the biochemical system responsible for carrying DHA into the brain. Perhaps alcoholics suffer this defect as well. If so, high levels of DHA accumulating in the blood would reflect an absence of DHA in the brain. If this theory is correct, suggests Hibbeln, higher than normal doses of omega-3 might reverse the trend, raising DHA levels not only in the blood but also in the brain.

Because we cannot yet measure omega-3 fatty acids in the human brain without invasive—and obviously destructive—techniques, Hibbeln's hypothesis cannot yet be tested directly. Moreover, his group did not assess the impact of EPA, a long-chain omega-3 oil that with DHA, might play a role in reducing violence and stress. In years to come, well-designed placebo-controlled studies involving both DHA and EPA should clarify the issues. Our group at McLean Hospital is currently developing noninvasive tests based on magnetic resonance imaging technology to provide direct measurements of omega-3 fatty acids in the brain.

The Omega Deficit and Violent Youth

With so much violence in our nation's schools, we may ask, why is this epidemic particularly rampant among the young? One answer comes from the science of brain imaging. Dr. Deborah Yurgelun-Todd, a neuropsychologist and brain imaging researcher at McLean Hospital, recently published a fascinating study, which revealed that young people may have immature frontal lobes. Responsible for impulse control, among other functions, the frontal lobes do not mature until the early twenties. With immature frontal lobes boosting impulsivity, it is possible that a deficiency of one or more omega-3 oils might be especially dangerous.

It is worth noting that mood-related problems in children and adolescents contain the potential for aggression and violence. For example, children who are manic or depressed may exhibit aggressive, risk-taking behavior. In certain types of attention deficit–hyperactivity disorder (ADHD), the hyperactivity and impulsivity characteristic of this disorder may lead to aggression. Substance abuse, which some researchers feel is often an attempt at self-medicating mood or ADHD symptoms, fits in this category too. Alcohol and drugs can lower inhibitions, increasing the potential for aggression and violence.

Along these lines, scientists at Purdue University have drawn a connection between omega-3 fatty acid deficit and temper tantrums, among other symptoms. To do the study, Laura J. Stevens and other researchers at Purdue recruited ninety-six boys, age six to twelve. The boys received health checkups, had blood tests, and went through a psychiatric evaluation. Those with greater levels of impulsivity were found to have low levels of the essential fatty acids, both omega-6 and omega-3, in their blood. It is possible that omega-3 deficiency in children is associated with deficiency in learning ability and visual processing. Especially significant was the prevalence of ADHD symptoms and temper tantrums in the low-omega group.

The New Pharmacology of Aggression

From "conduct disorder" to "intermittent explosive disorder," many psychiatric diagnoses with an aggressive component are treated with drugs. If violence appears to be part of another, overarching disorder—bipolar disorder, for instance—then psychiatrists generally treat the underlying problem and hope the violent behavior decreases.

But things are often more complex. Patients may have more than one diagnosis—a major "biological" disorder like bipolar disorder, for instance, along with other psychiatric or psychological illnesses, such as a longstanding personality disorder based on childhood neglect or trauma. These disorders arise, moreover, within the context of a genetic vulnerability and are also highly dependent on the age of the individual at the time of the abuse. However, not everyone raised in a violent, abusive, neglectful home will become ill, just as not every Vietnam combat veteran came home with post-traumatic stress disorder.

In light of this, medications have emerged specifically to take the edge off explosive anger and rage. These medications include the anticonvulsant drugs gabapentin (Neurontin) and divalproex sodium (Depakote), the beta-blockers propranolol (Inderal) and others, the conventional and the newer "atypical" antipsychotic agents, and many others. These treatments are most effective when combined with psychotherapy and with attention paid to social and environmental change.

The latest research suggests that supplements of omega-3 fatty acids may also be effective at countering some aggressive behavior and helping us deal with stress. Although the implications are powerful, much more work must be done to prove that omega-3 fatty acid supplements can reduce a tendency to violence. We await the results of future studies in our nation's schools and prisons, and hope that at least part of the answer may be as simple as an omega-3 fatty acid.

....

9

....

Omega-3 Deficiency and Attention Deficit: The Case for a Connection

∽ One of the most prevalent psychiatric illnesses of childhood, attention deficit–hyperactivity disorder, seems to have burst on the modern scene. Virtually unheard of—and literally un-named—even fifty years ago, ADHD is today so commonplace it afflicts nearly five of every one hundred schoolchildren (and, say the experts, possibly as many adults). The increased rate of ADHD diagnosis appears to be far in excess of merely increased recognition of the disorder. Although ADHD comes with a range of symptoms, those with the disorder are intelligent, yet most often have difficulty paying attention, listening to instructions, or completing tasks. Children with ADHD often fidget, squirm, and disrupt their classmates; some find it impossible to deal with unstructured settings at all.

Mild forms of ADHD can add challenge and difficulty to the most ordinary tasks, from balancing a checkbook to completing a homework assignment, despite a high IQ. As Internet bulletin boards and the popular press make abundantly clear, untreated ADHD may destroy lives—severely compromising school performance, shattering self-esteem, turning a family into a war zone, or making it difficult to find and keep friends. ADHD seems to prevent its sufferers from having full access to their abilities by both a Parkinson-like difficulty with initiating action, combined with a restlessness that prevents successful focus on the task at hand.

DSM-IV Criteria for ADHD in Children or Adults

To meet the diagnostic criteria, symptoms must be present for at least six months, with onset before age seven. There are three essential varieties of ADHD: one characterized by inattention, another by hyperactivity, and a third that combines the symptoms of both.

Inattention

1. Often fails to give close attention to details or makes careless mistakes in schoolwork, work, or other activities.
2. Often has difficulty sustaining attention in tasks or play activities.
3. Often does not seem to listen when spoken to directly.
4. Often does not follow through on instructions and fails to finish schoolwork, chores, or duties in the workplace (not due to being obstructive or failure to understand instructions).
5. Often has difficulty organizing tasks and activities.
6. Often avoids, dislikes, or is reluctant to engage in tasks that require sustained mental effort (such as schoolwork or homework).
7. Often loses things necessary for tasks or activities (e.g., toys, school assignments, pencils, books, or tools).
8. Is often easily distracted by extraneous stimuli.
9. Is often forgetful in daily activities.

Hyperactivity-Impulsivity

1. Often fidgets with hands or feet or squirms in seat.
2. Often leaves his or her seat in the classroom or in other situations in which remaining seated is expected.
3. Often runs about or climbs excessively in situations in which it is inappropriate (in adolescents or adults, they might be limited to subjective feelings of restlessness).
4. Often has difficulty playing or engaging in leisure activities quietly.
5. Is often on the go or often acts as if driven by a motor.
6. Often talks excessively.
7. Often blurts out answers before questions have been completed.
8. Often has difficulty awaiting turn.
9. Often interrupts or intrudes on others.

Remember, according to Children and Adults with Attention Deficit/Hyperactivity Disorder (CHADD), the national organization for ADHD, all children may be overly active at times. Their attention spans may be short, and they may act without thinking. However, a child who does seem more active than others the same age; is notoriously forgetful, disorganized, and always losing things; can't stay seated or quiet in class; blurts out answers instead of waiting to be called on; pays more attention to the traffic in the hall than to the events in the classroom; and behaves aggressively or impulsively, should be evaluated for ADHD.

Determining if a child has ADHD is a multifaceted process. Many biological and psychological problems can contribute to symptoms similar to those exhibited by children with ADHD. For example, bipolar disorder, anxiety, depression, and certain types of learning disabilities may cause similar symptoms.

A comprehensive evaluation is necessary to establish a

diagnosis, rule out other causes and determine the presence or absence of concurrent conditions. Such an evaluation should include a clinical assessment of academic, social, and emotional function and developmental abilities. Additional tests may include intelligence testing, measures of attention span and parent and teacher rating scales. A medical exam by a physician is also important.

Diagnosing ADHD in an adult requires an examination of childhood, academic, and behavioral history. The problems need to have started in childhood but persist into adulthood. Fifty percent of children with ADHD continue to have symptoms into adulthood. Adults tend to lose the hyperactivity symptoms, but often retain the inattention and impulsive behaviors.

A Treatable Disorder

In what has been a godsend for those with ADHD, the disorder has turned out to be among the most treatable of the psychiatric ills. In some 70 percent of those diagnosed, the modern arsenal of medication—including stimulants like Ritalin and Dexedrine, and a range of antidepressants, from Wellbutrin to impramine—can address the more incapacitating symptoms. As with other psychiatric disorders, successful drug treatment suggests a biochemical origin, yet the most effective treatments involve combinations of medication and behavioral therapy.

The leap was first made in 1937, with the serendipitous discovery that the stimulant drug Benzedrine could dramatically reduce the symptoms of hyperactive children. Physicians later found that Ritalin and Cylert, two other stimulants, were dramatically effective as well. The findings were counterintuitive: logic suggested that hyperactive children were already overstimulated and that stimulant medication would push them further along the curve. Because the opposite occurred, researchers believed that a complex biochemical disturbance was at play.

Researchers have been trying to nail down the brain chemistry of ADHD ever since. The first clue came with the discovery that stimulants increase the activity of two specific chemicals in the brain: the neurotransmitters norepinephrine and dopamine. It seemed logical to conclude that ADHD resulted when these neurotransmitters were in short supply. Yet attempts to document this through biochemical analysis have fallen short. This is likely because the mechanism is more complex. Among the confusing issues is that medications that influence norepinephrine and dopamine also alter serotonin and other neurotransmitters in the brain.

Researchers do know, however, through PET (positron emission tomography) scans of the brain, that those with the disorder show lower levels of activity in specific regions of the brain. The most recent imaging studies show that three brain regions controlling attention and behavior—the prefrontal cortex, part of the basal ganglia, and the vermis region of the cerebellum—are significantly smaller in children with ADHD.

Although much still remains unknown, it is likely that ADHD resides largely in the genes. ADHD runs in families, frequently going back generations. Perhaps most convincing is a study showing that if an identical twin has ADHD, the other is between eleven and eighteen times more likely to have it than a non-twin sibling.

Experts still do not know just what causes ADHD, and they are perplexed by the precipitous rise of ADHD during the past fifty years in the industrialized West.

Even with these gaps in our knowledge, however, those on the front lines of treatment know that the correct pharmacological mix can be remarkably helpful while lack of medication may consign children to lives of difficulty and distress. Perhaps that is why those specialists have been so resistant to voices outside the mainstream, ranging from those who say the disorder is invented to biofeedback folks who contend that symptoms may be abated by controlling one's own mind. Barraged by treatments du jour, from allergy shots to homeopathy, ADHD specialists have seen dozens of bogus "therapies" come and go.

Yet the current standard of care, though effective, is far from perfect. Pharmacological and behavioral treatments for ADHD do not usually eliminate all symptoms and may cause side effects such as sleeplessness and weight loss. However, effective treatment can allow individuals access to their abilities and intelligence, making huge differences in their self-esteem and capacity to function in the world.

A Domino Theory: One Deficit Begets Another

Why are there so many cases of ADHD today? The answer may come from a theory circulating among scientists studying lipids and their impact on the brain: the explosion of ADHD in a generation of American children midway through the twentieth century might possibly be rooted in the parallel deficit of a vital brain nutrient, the omega-3 fatty acids.

For a core group of lipid scientists, the first inkling that omega-3 deficit might be connected to attention deficit emerged with the popularization of ADHD itself. By 1981, as the problems of ADHD children gained increasing attention in the press, researchers noticed the similarities between ADHD and omega-3 fatty acid deficiency. Both groups reported excess thirst and the increased need to urinate; both had greater frequency of dry hair and skin, and, most striking, some 40 percent of those with ADHD had low levels of omega-3 fatty acids in the blood.

The case for the connection between these two seeming disparate conditions starts with studies of animals. Rats on diets deficient in omega-3 fatty acids are less able to learn in new environments. Monkeys fed a pre- and postnatal diet deficient in omega-3 fatty acids drink more fluids and excrete more urine and feces. Caged monkeys on a diet low in omega-3 fats are more likely to display stereotyped, repetitive behaviors and levels of locomotion far in excess of counterparts fed healthy levels of the essential fatty acids.

Rats with Attention Deficit

A 1998 study from the University of South Florida College of Medicine established the extraordinary fact that rat pups given fish oil supplements showed delays in neurodevelopment compared to a group fed corn oil. On the face of it, this might seem to argue *against* omega-3 fats as nutrients for the brain. But the particular attribute measured as a sign of neurodevelopment was the auditory startle response. As any ADHD expert knows, the threshold to reaction—including time to startle—is lower, not higher, in those diagnosed with ADHD.

The Florida findings are especially fascinating in light of the latest theory put forth by ADHD researcher Russell Barkley, Director of Psychology and Professor of Psychiatry and Neurology at the University of Massachusetts Medical Center in Worcester. Barkley holds that the key to the disorder is an inability to inhibit responses to stimuli from the world. "We are finding ADHD is not a disorder of attention per se, as had long been assumed," he recently wrote. "Rather it arises as a developmental failure in the brain circuitry that underlies inhibition and self-control. This loss of self-control in turn impairs other important brain functions crucial for maintaining attention."

A series of rat studies from France, meanwhile, focused on omega-3 fatty acid deficiency and its impact on the neurotransmitters in ADHD. Analyzing the frontal cortex, the scientists found that when compared with controls, animals deprived of omega-3 oils had significantly less dopamine and dopamine receptors along with more serotonin receptors, a possible indicator of less available serotonin.

How did the neurotransmitter profile relate to behavior associated with ADHD? Based on prior studies, the scientists already knew that rats with omega-3 deficiency and abnormal levels of dopamine and serotonin score lower on tests of learning and memory. Yet learning and memory are not really the qualities directly compromised in human ADHD, where it is the ability to pay attention, not remember or learn, that is the issue at hand. A better measure, reasoned the French scientists, would be distractibility. Would rats on a diet rich in omega-3 oils be more likely to pay attention and complete tasks?

To measure distractibility, the scientists trained rats to move through a runway tube from starting point to finish line, providing sugared water as their reward at the end. As a distraction, they extended a second perpendicular runway midway through the body of the first. The notion was that the most attentive rats would ignore the extra runway and move straight to their reward; as distractibility increased, rats would dally for increasingly longer periods in the auxiliary setup before turning around and moving on.

The findings seemed to mirror human models of ADHD in significant ways. Rats with diets deficient in omega-3 fatty acids were most distractible and took longest to reach the goal; it was notable that, as occurs with many ADHD children, symptoms of distractibility decreased with age.

The Human Evidence

Although controlled studies of children deficient in omega-3 oils have been far more difficult to orchestrate, the clinical findings match the results gleaned from animals in the lab. In 1987, for instance, researchers studying forty-eight hyperactive children showed not only that they had more health and learning problems than children without hyperactivity—entirely expected—but also that they were thirstier and urinated more frequently. The hyperactive children also had significantly lower blood levels of two omega-6 oils (arachidonic and dihomogammalinolenic acids) and one omega-3 oil, the brain-building DHA, perhaps signifying generally poor nutrition.

The key work connecting omega-3 deficit and attention deficit has been done over the past few years by John R. Burgess and his team at Purdue University. In one study, the group compared lipids in the blood of fifty-three ADHD boys to a control group of forty-three boys without ADHD. The ADHD boys had significantly lower levels of the essential fatty acids arachidonic (omega-6), EPA (omega-3), and DHA (omega-3). Overall, 40 percent of the ADHD boys in the study also had the symptoms of omega-3 deficiency, including increased urination and thirst. Compare this to the 9 percent of boys without ADHD who exhibited these symptoms.

In a parallel study, apparently in the same ninety-six boys (aged six to twelve), Burgess found that those with low levels of omega-3 fatty acids in the blood were more likely to have the behavior problems that are characteristic of ADHD, whether or not they were actually diagnosed with the disorder. "We are trying to find potential causes of ADHD so that nutritional treatments can be developed," said Burgess, who is an assistant professor of food and nutrition. This was an important study, and it provides direction for future research.

Treatments for the Future

Even if omega-3 fatty acid deficit turns out to be a factor in the development of some cases of ADHD, it is a leap from there to the notion that fatty fish or fish oil supplements might address the symptoms. Burgess, for instance, found that even when ADHD children are fed more omega-3 fatty acids than controls, they end up with less in their system. "We still don't know why some children have low levels of omega-3 fatty acids in their blood while others do not," Burgess says. "The body does not need huge quantities of omega-3 fatty acids, and it is possible that those with ADHD cannot process what they need from the foods they eat."

To answer this question, Burgess and others are testing omega-3 fatty acid supplements on ADHD children. In a study based at the Mayo Medical School in Rochester, Minnesota, and Baylor College of Medicine in Houston, Texas, researchers are providing sixty-three ADHD children with supplements of pure DHA or placebo and testing them for any decrease of inattention, impulsivity, or hyperactivity. While researchers are merely adding supplements to stimulant medication in the first part of the study, the second part calls for halving the stimulant dose (in those on supplements) to see whether DHA can reduce the need for stimulant medication. Burgess is testing supplements on a population of fifty ADHD children who also have symptoms of omega-3 deficiency to see whether symptoms of one or both disorders will subside. Even if DHA fails to improve the symptoms of ADHD, EPA (the other long-chain omega-3 fatty acid) requires testing. EPA and DHA appear to have very different properties in the brain.

While it will be some time before scientists have definitive answers about the omega-3 connection in ADHD, preliminary research suggests that trying DHA or EPA may be useful.

10

Treating Schizophrenia with Omega-3 Oils

✐ Of the common mental illnesses, schizophrenia is one of the most devastating. It generally strikes people in their teens or early twenties, destroying hopes for a normal academic, social, and vocational future. Afflicting some 1 percent of the population, or one out of every one hundred people, it is marked by severe disorganization, disintegration of personality, and distorted perceptions of reality, including bizarre thoughts and hallucinations. Those with this disease often exhibit bizarre delusions and may believe they are controlled by brain implants or aliens, or that they are the reincarnation of some long-dead figure like George Washington, Cleopatra, or King Henry VIII. They may see entities and hear voices that threaten them, instruct them to perform bizarre rituals, or sustain running commentaries on their lives. If untreated, in the most severe cases of schizophrenia, the afflicted may seem incoherent or "catatonic," remaining in a stuporous state in which they are mute and immobile. Effective antipsychotic medicines are available that usually only partially relieve the symptoms. Recently, the omega-3 fatty acid EPA has been shown to be a powerful adjunct.

Psychiatrists diagnose schizophrenia according to the standards set forth in the *Diagnostic and Statistical Manual of Mental Disorders*, 4th edition (DSM-IV). The symptoms fall into two categories: "positive" symptoms, including hallucinations, delusions, and agitation (common in the early stages of schizophrenia), and "negative" symptoms, including social withdrawal, cognitive decline, and apathy (characteristic of advanced schizophrenia).

DSM-IV Criteria for Schizophrenia

A. *Characteristic symptoms:* Two (or more) of the following, each present for a significant portion of time during a one-month period (or less if successfully treated).
1. delusions
2. hallucinations
3. disorganized speech (e.g., frequent derailment or incoherence)
4. grossly disorganized or catatonic behavior
5. negative symptoms, i.e., affective flattening, alogia, or avolition

Note: Only one criterion A symptom is required if delusions are bizarre or hallucinations consist of a voice keeping up a running commentary on the person's behavior or thoughts, or two or more voices conversing with each other.

B. *Social/occupational dysfunction:* For a significant portion of the time since the onset of the disturbance, one or more major areas of functioning, such as work, interpersonal relations, or self-care are markedly below the level achieved prior to the onset (or when the onset is in childhood or adolescence, failure to achieve the expected level of interpersonal, academic, or occupational achievement).

C. *Duration:* Continual signs of the disturbance persist for at least six months. This six-month period must include at least one month of symptoms (or less if successfully treated) that meet criterion A (i.e., active-phase symptoms) and may include periods of prodromal or residual symptoms. During these prodromal or residual periods, the signs of the disturbance might be manifested by only negative symptoms or two or more symptoms listed in criterion A present in attenuated form (e.g., odd beliefs, unusual perceptual experiences).

D. *Schizoaffective and mood disorder exclusion:* Schizoaffective disorder and mood disorder with psychotic features have been ruled out because either (1) no major depressive, manic, or mixed episodes have occurred concurrently with the active-phase symptoms or (2) if mood episodes have occurred during active-phase symptoms, their total duration has been brief relative to the duration of the active and residual periods.

E. *Substance/general medical condition exclusion:* The disturbance is not due to the direct physiological effects of a substance (e.g., a drug of abuse, a medication) or a general medical condition.

The clinical course of schizophrenia tends to be chronic, unremitting, and progressive. The state of the art treatment had been the class of antipsychotic drugs called the neuroleptics, developed in the 1950s. Including such well-known brands as Thorazine, Haldol, Stelazine, and Trilafon, the neuroleptics were fairly successful in relieving the positive symptoms of schizophrenia. Flush with the power of these new medications, and in conjunction with the political and economic forces of the time, American state mental hospitals of the 1950s and 1960s virtually emptied their wards, releasing previously untreatable patients with schizophrenia to the care of outpatient mental health centers within the community. Nearly fifty years later, at the turn of the millennium, this "solution" has left a national disaster in its wake. Without appropriate support from outpatient facilities to which they were assigned and with increasing cuts in funding over the years, large numbers of these patients now roam the streets. Off their medication and constituting a large segment of the nation's homeless, they are hungry, disoriented, alone, and neglected.

Newer, safe, and more effective medications have rendered the older neuroleptics virtually obsolete. These so-called atypical antipsychotic agents—including Risperdal (risperidone), Zyprexa (olanzapine), Seroquel (quetiapine), and Clozaril (clozapine)—treat the positive symptoms as well as (or better in the case of Clozaril) conventional antipsychotic agents, and are superior in reducing the negative symptoms. The atypicals are also safer (with the exception of clozapine) because, by and large, they do not cause the neurological symptoms and potentially life-threatening side effects of the earlier drugs.

Despite such advances, the plight of the patient with schizophrenia in the United States grows worse. At the request of the *Los Angeles Times*, the California Department of Mental Health recently asked seven counties to dig through their records to determine the fate of 2,509 men and women released from state hospitals in 1991, the year that the state ceded control of $1 billion in funds for care of this group to the counties. Half of those released in this bureaucratic shuffle were doing fairly well, the state learned, but the outcome for the rest was bleak. At least 6 percent had died, some violently. Hundreds failed to succeed on the outside, with at least 9 percent back in state hospitals and about 15 percent relegated to cheaper alternatives: privately run, locked nursing homes for the mentally ill, some with reputations for patient neglect and abuse. Hundreds more are unaccounted for, and 11 percent have not had contact with a state mental health worker since 1996. Los Angeles County alone had 948 patients in state mental hospitals in 1991. Of the 933 released, 27 percent had been jailed and 20 percent had been homeless at least once. Replayed across the nation, the California story is the American story as well.

The Eight-Country Study

Hoping to better understand the course and outcome of this debilitating mental illness, the United Nations' World Health Organization (WHO) conducted a long-term study of schizophrenia in eight countries worldwide. Its findings were twofold: the frequency of the disease is consistent at 1 percent of the population across all nations, and the prognosis for patients with schizophrenia is worse in the United States than in developing nations like Nigeria and India, despite the availability in the United States of modern antipsychotic drugs.

The discrepancy was perplexing to two Danish scientists, the husband and wife team of O. Christensen and E. Christensen. Seeking an explanation, they noticed that the eight nations in the WHO study differed not only in terms of outcome for schizophrenia but also in terms of dietary fat. Countries with the worst outcomes tended to consume mostly saturated fat; those with the best outcomes obtained most of their fat from fruit, nuts, and fish.

To quantify the difference, the Christensens compared the WHO findings to data gleaned from the Food and Agriculture Organization, another branch of the UN. Placing the two sets of data side by side, they confirmed their observation: across the board, nations consuming the highest levels of saturated fat had the worst outcomes from schizophrenia while those consuming the highest levels of vegetable and fish fats—especially those rich in omega-3 fatty acids—had the best outcomes. So powerful was the relationship that fat consumption could account for 85 percent of the differences between nations. When the Christensens looked at omega-3 fatty acids alone, the correlation was even more dramatic, and strikingly similar to the findings on depression and heart disease described earlier in this book.

Membranes on Strike

The findings from the Christensen and WHO study might be best explained by the theories of lipid pioneer David Horrobin, M.D., a neuroendocrinologist devoted to pharmacological research and products based on essential fatty acids. Researching and writing about essential fatty acids and the brain for nearly two decades, Dr. Horrobin has long espoused the so-called membrane phospholipid hypothesis of schizophrenia. According to this theory, patients with negative symptoms of schizophrenia—those who are withdrawn, incoherent, or catatonic—are thought to suffer from defective cell membranes and an abnormality in lipid biochemistry. Stemming from some genetic alteration, this defect may prevent membranes from incorporating essential fatty acids. Schizophrenia, Horrobin believes, is the tragic result.

Although mainstream psychiatry has long considered this theory controversial, various research findings support it:

- In schizophrenic patients, pathological changes in many neurotransmitter systems suggest a global disorder—something that would make sense if membranes were defective throughout the entire brain.
- Brain scans using magnetic resonance imaging technology show that schizophrenic patients—whether on drug therapy or not—break down phospholipids at an abnormal rate.
- Blood platelets from schizophrenic patients incorporate unsaturated fatty acids at reduced rates.
- Schizophrenic patients with negative symptoms have lower levels of the essential fatty acids in red blood cells than those with positive symptoms.
- Air expired by schizophrenics shows significantly increased levels of the gas pentane, consistent with increased breakdown of essential fatty acids.

The (Fatty) Acid Test

The acid test for any medical theory or treatment is data from clinical studies—preferably those that are double-blind, placebo-controlled, and reviewed by other scientists in the same field. While we await the publication of just such studies for omega-3 fats and schizophrenia, we are encouraged by the apparent dramatic success of more preliminary work.

At the forefront of the new research is Malcolm Peet, head of the Omega-3 Mental Health Research Group at the University of Sheffield in the United Kingdom. Established specifically to investigate the phospholipid hypothesis of mental health disorders, the Sheffield team has thus far tested EPA and DHA supplements for schizophrenia in three different studies.

In one study, twenty schizophrenic patients received daily fish oil supplements high in EPA and DHA. At the end of the six-week trial, the researchers found increased levels of omega-3 fatty acids in these patients' red blood cell membranes, along with improvements in both positive and negative symptoms of schizophrenia—though only measurements of negative symptoms proved statistically significant.

In another study, Peet and staff examined among schizophrenic patients the effect of being breast-fed as a baby. Using carefully matched control subjects, the researchers found that only 44 percent of schizophrenic patients had been breast-fed for more than four weeks, relative to 67 percent of the control group. Because infant formula is deficient in omega-3 fatty acids compared to breast milk, bottle feeding without omega-3 supplementation may exacerbate a metabolic imbalance already in place.

The Sheffield group has also conducted the only double-blind, placebo-controlled study on omega-3 fatty acids and schizophrenia to date. This preliminary trial compared an EPA-enriched oil, a DHA-enriched oil, and a corn-oil placebo in the treatment of forty-five schizophrenic patients resistant to treatment with conventional antipsychotic medication. Study participants stayed on their antipsychotic drugs during the three-month trial period, but were given omega-3 supplements as well.

The scientists were surprised to find that EPA alone was effective. They had expected to find that DHA, so prevalent in cell membranes, would result in the biggest improvement, but when the study ended and the data were analyzed, the Sheffield team found that EPA was associated with an impressive 24 percent improvement in positive symptoms compared to almost 14 percent for controls and 3 percent for DHA.

The Sheffield group used blood levels of the different omega-3s in an attempt to explain their findings. They found that EPA in red blood cell membranes of the EPA-supplemented patients increased an astounding forty-five times while DHA in the membranes of DHA-supplemented patients only doubled. The discrepancy may stem from the important role of DHA in cell membranes: the human body may simply hold on to DHA more tightly than other lipids (including EPA) even in the face of dietary omega-3 fatty acid deficiency. If this is the case, EPA would be in shorter supply than DHA, and cells would incorporate EPA at a greater rate to make up for the greater deficiency.

Peet and colleagues say this line of research bolsters the membrane phospholipid hypothesis of schizophrenia. Schizophrenia has already been associated with elevated levels of an enzyme that breaks down membranes. The efficacy of EPA could be explained if future studies reveal it to reverse the action of this enzyme. There may be alternative explanations because EPA has many functions in the brain that we are just beginning to understand.

The Omega Cure

Whatever the ultimate explanation, the Sheffield findings have encouraged other researchers to test EPA in the clinical setting as well. Reports from the field are dramatic, and reveal a need for greater study of EPA.

Researchers at the Imperial College School of Medicine in London, for instance, decided to try EPA therapy on a thirty-one-year-old patient who consistently refused antipsychotic medications due to fear of side effects. Suffering from daily auditory hallucinations and a complex delusional system since his late teenage years, the patient had, at the time of treatment, begun to show negative symptoms like social withdrawal as well. Reporting in the *Archives of General Psychiatry*, Basant K. Puri, Robert Steiner, and Alexandra Richardson of the Imperial College say their patient improved so dramatically following two months of EPA therapy that he went into remission. "We believe it is unlikely that this represented either a spontaneous remission or a placebo response," the group writes. "The patient's clinical profile had remained essentially unchanged during the two previous years, and prior to this there is no evidence of spontaneous remission or an episodic quality to his illness."

Psychiatrists at the University of Baroda in India have been collaborating with the Sheffield group. Although the Indian diet is naturally higher in omega-3 fatty acids and Indians suffer less severe forms of schizophrenia than in the West, the disease is still a problem of enormous proportion in an impoverished nation where there is a paucity of medical care. Hoping to find a better treatment, the Baroda researchers conducted a pilot study of ten schizophrenic patients who responded only poorly to conventional antipsychotic drugs. After twelve weeks on an EPA supplement, the Baroda patients experienced a 25 percent reduction in symptoms, identical to their British counterparts.

The Antioxidant Boost

Hope of developing a natural treatment for schizophrenia is strengthened by recent evidence that vitamins C and E might boost the EPA effect. In research out of the Medical College of Georgia in Augusta, psychiatric researcher Dr. Sahebarao P. Mahadik has found that patients with schizophrenia contain very high blood levels of biochemical markers of what lipid scientists call lipid peroxidation—the oxidation, or chemical destruction, of fatty acids by oxygen and other highly reactive chemicals, such as free radicals, in the body. When membrane fatty acids become oxidized, they are chemically deactivated; they no longer function in their original role and are eliminated from the body. Excessive lipid peroxides can also damage cell membranes.

Because the omega-3 chemical structure is exceptionally fragile, EPA and DHA are highly susceptible to oxidation. If the intake of dietary omega-3 fatty acids is inadequate, oxidative destruction could hasten an omega-3 deficiency.

In a series of early studies, Mahadik added the common antioxidant vitamins C and E to conventional antipsychotic treatments for schizophrenia and some other associated disorders. His results suggest that the patients who received adequate amounts of vitamin C—at least 1,000 milligrams per day—and vitamin E—at least 800 IU (International Units) per day—fared better than the patients who did not receive these supplements.

Mahadik believes that both antioxidant vitamins are necessary. Vitamin E is soluble in fat. Since the cell membrane is made mostly of fat, vitamin E stays in or near the cell membrane. There, it can use its antioxidant powers to reduce or even prevent the oxidation of the incorporated fatty acids, including the omega-3s.

Vitamin C is also crucial, he notes, because it is water soluble. It is best at acting in the watery cytoplasm inside the cell, as well as in the mitochondria, the cellular energy factories, that are located in the cytoplasm. Fatty acids are oxidized by mitochondrial enzymes, which ultimately convert them to carbon dioxide, water, and energy for use by the cell. Normal oxidation of fats is a necessary part of cellular functioning, but abnormal or excessive oxidation of crucial fatty acids, such as the omega-3s, may produce disease states. Vitamin C dissolved in the cytoplasm of the cell may prevent or reduce excessive essential fatty acid oxidation in the mitochondria. Another theory is that vitamin C's main action involves replenishing vitamin E stores, which become depleted as vitamin E performs its antioxidant function.

Based on his research, Mahadik suggests that the therapeutic benefit of EPA might be enhanced with additional supplements of vitamins C and E. If confirmed, the antioxidant boost could extend beyond schizophrenia into bipolar disorder, major depression, and the other psychiatric and medical disorders where the omega-3 fatty acids have been shown to be beneficial.

Awaiting Final Word

The current findings require confirmation, but nonetheless suggest that omega-3 fatty acids, particularly EPA, may have an important role in schizophrenia and other psychiatric conditions. Not only may EPA be a potentially effective antipsychotic agent in its own right, but it may also enhance the therapeutic value of conventional antipsychotic drugs. With vitamins C and E as further adjuvants, a natural and safe breakthrough in the treatment of schizophrenia may be at hand.

11

Memory and Cognition: The Omega Boost

෴ Over the past decade, researchers have documented the broad-based role of omega-3 deficit in heart disease, immune problems, and psychiatric disorders, among other illnesses. But what about those without a clinical deficit—with omega-3 fatty acid levels that are adequate, even ideal? Will providing still more—supplemental omega-3 oils, above and beyond the nutritional guidelines—cause problems? Or will such boosters push us still further along the curve of mental sharpness and health?

In most medical specialties and scientific disciplines, the issue of health enhancement is unstudied. The use of "megadose" nutrients, vitamins, and supplements remains largely unexplored scientifically and can be dangerous with certain vitamins, such as A, D, or E. Anecdotal or even fictional reports of enhanced bodily or mental functioning from such high-dose supplements are widespread. Literature and Web sites from disreputable firms often make wild and unsubstantiated claims. The dramatic promise of enhanced health sells products. If we are free from heart disease and cancer, after all, why not be content? However, the quest for an edge can be keen, particularly in areas like mood, memory, and learning. Natural food pundits have advocated ginkgo biloba, ginseng, and other herbs to stoke the engines of cognition. However, two of the leading natural candidates for cognitive sharpening may be the long-chain omega-3 fatty acids, EPA and DHA.

Numerous studies document the role of omega-3 fatty acids in the development of the human brain. Animals and humans lacking these fatty acids during gestation and the first years of life score lower on IQ tests and a range of cognitive benchmarks. Convincing studies have traced omega-3 fatty acid deficits to reduced scores on measures of attention across different species, from humans to mice. Now, it turns out, the latest work may extend these findings; a *surplus* of omega-3 oils may possibly sharpen attention and enhance learning, even in those who had appropriate omega-3 levels before the studies began.

Smart Mice

The first evidence comes from studies in Japan of mice. In an initial experiment, the researchers studied a group of prematurely aging mice they called SAM-P because they were genetically "senescence *prone*," (wired to age prematurely). The SAM-P mice showed age-related impairments in memory and learning far earlier than normal mice. Yet when fed perilla oil (from the perilla plant, which contains high levels of the omega-3 fatty acid alpha-linolenic acid), the SAM-P animals were able to learn significantly more effectively than their genetically similar SAM-P siblings fed safflower oil (a source of omega-6 fatty acids). The improved profile for learning with the omega-3 supplement led the researchers to wonder just what kind of mechanism was operating. Had the ability to learn and remember really improved or were the mice merely performing on target thanks to a positive emotional state, including reduced anxiety?

To find out, they decided to test SAM-R (for "senescence-resistant") strains of mice, which do not show age-related deterioration of learning and memory. The team again fed the mice either perilla oil or safflower oil over the course of two generations, and then tested them for hyperactivity, exploratory behavior, and learning, among other traits. The researchers found that the SAM-R mice fed safflower oil (omega-6) were more hyperactive than those on perilla oil (omega-3) but scored lower when it came to actual exploration of the environment. The more hyperactive the mice were, the less likely they were to display normal, adaptive exploratory behavior.

Mice supplemented with omega-3 oils were also better learners. In one experimental setup, mice were trained to push a lever in response to cues of light or dark; correct responses were rewarded with pellets of food. As the test went on, the mice given omega-3 supplements made significantly fewer mistakes. They were also better at responding when the conditions of the experiment changed. When scientists stopped delivering the pellet reward after numerous trials, the omega-3-supplemented mice noticed the change and adjusted their behavior accordingly, while the safflower-oil-fed, unsupplemented mice did not.

Fat for Thought

Human studies parallel the findings in mice and rats. The most compelling evidence comes from psychologist David Benton, a professor at the University of Wales in the United Kingdom. Benton has found that low-fat diets in general often impede reaction times, memory, and cognitive skills. In a study of 9,003 British participants, for instance, he found that people who consumed more fat, including saturated fat, could react more rapidly to stimulation. In a related study of 153 women, he found lower cholesterol levels—known to lower risk of heart disease—were nonetheless also associated with slower reaction time. Finally, in a recent controlled study of 285 healthy young women, he found that vigilance—attention to task—was significantly enhanced for those on 400 milligrams of DHA a day versus those taking a placebo sugar pill.

Most researchers have traditionally focused on DHA, not EPA, in studies of brain function since DHA is heavily incorporated into the cell membranes of neurons. But fish oil often contains more EPA than DHA. EPA is both incorporated into cell membranes and circulated in the bloodstream, bathing all parts of the body, including brain tissue. Also, the body of someone who is deficient in omega-3 fatty acids will hold on tightly to DHA while EPA levels continue to drop. It is important to remember that even though less EPA is incorporated into membranes than DHA, the EPA that is in the membrane is highly active and has a rapid turnover rate.

For those taking omega-3 supplements, it is the rise in EPA that often correlates with response. There is a growing amount of scientific data suggesting that EPA may be the crucial omega-3 fatty acid in sustaining mood, cardiovascular health, and more. At this point in our knowledge of the omega-3 fatty acids, we have not determined if EPA, DHA, or both are the crucial components of fish oil for mental health. Are they redundant or do they have independent, distinct actions?

Rejuvenating the Brain

The most exciting finding, it turns out, may be new hope for revving the engine of the aging brain. As the senescent-prone mice illustrate, aging impairs not just memory but also the rapidity and accuracy of thought. Gerontologists on the trail of cognitive decline in humans have focused on a few biochemical factors, including polyunsaturated fats (omega-6 and omega-3 fatty acids).

To test the theory that omega-3 fatty acids keep the brain active longer, a team of Dutch scientists studied cognition in a group of men aged sixty-nine to eighty-nine. The men were part of what is known as the Zutphen Elderly Study, which looked at risk factors for chronic diseases in men who live in Zutphen, a town in the eastern part of the Netherlands. Interestingly, the Zutphen Elderly Study is a continuation of the original Zutphen

Study, initiated in 1960 as the Dutch contribution to the famed Seven Countries Study that examined nutrients and disease across a range of cultures. This aging group of men with a wealth of health data and well-documented nutritional profiles was ideal for investigating the impact of omega-3 fatty acids on life-long maintenance of brain function.

With that in mind, the researchers set out to interview the Zutphen men, documenting their dietary habits in the spring of 1985 and then assessing their cognitive skills in 1990 and again in 1993. The original group consisted of 1,266 men; 555 subjects (44 percent) were still alive in 1985. However, only 342 men (27 percent) were available for the final cognitive assessment in 1993.

The results painted a sobering picture of the aging brain. Thirty-two percent of the surviving subjects were cognitively impaired in 1990, with the oldest and least educated the most impaired of all. The scientists found that the cognitive decline did not alter diet in these men; they ate the same general diet after impairment as before. When the data were analyzed, it became apparent that certain foods—including margarine, butter, baking fat, sauces, and cheese—placed subjects at especially high risk for later cognitive impairment.

The connection between cognitive impairment and fatty acid intake was especially striking: the average intake of total fat and certain polyunsaturated fatty acids (especially linoleic acid, an omega-6 oil) was higher in subjects with cognitive impairment while the intake of fish, EPA, DHA, and total energy was low. Stated another way, high consumption of fish was associated with less cognitive impairment. This makes sense because high levels of the omega-6 arachidonic acid can be neurotoxic. Surprisingly, there was no detectable relationship between lower cognitive impairment and consumption of any of the antioxidants (such as vitamins C and E) thought to protect the brain.

The protective powers of omega-3 fats may go far beyond the normal cognitive deficits of aging. New studies suggest that the omega-3s may at least partially protect us against the onslaught of debilitating brain illnesses like Alzheimer's or the permanent damage that results when, due to stroke or other vascular insults, we experience a temporary halt in the supply of blood to the brain. Japanese scientists, for instance, have shown that daily DHA supplements reduced the amount of brain damage that rats suffered after blood flow to the brain was temporarily blocked (an animal model of stroke). The researchers speculate that daily supplements of DHA taken over a period of weeks or months might reduce risk of brain damage and cognitive-spatial deficits in the aftermath of stroke. Should this be the case, candidates for this prophylactic therapy may be those with hypertension or other risk factors for stroke.

Balanced Brains

Despite these findings, a call for caution is necessary, especially for those who have no deficit or disease, and are simply seeking a boost. The latest studies reveal that when it comes to learning, adding omega-3 fatty acids to the diet without appropriate calories from omega-6 may have an adverse effect. This crucial caveat comes from scientists at Bar-Ilan University and Hillel Yaffe Hospital in Israel who have zeroed in on the specific ratio of omega-3 to omega-6 fatty acids required for optimum learning in rats.

To test rat learning, the Israeli researchers filled a circular tank with water and powdered milk. Rats swimming within were unable to see a slightly submerged inner escape platform due to the opacity of the milky water, but could navigate by referencing a view of the surrounding room, visible from the tank's periphery. The question at hand was this: would different dosages of the omega-3 and omega-6 oils alter rats' learning, including their ability to find the escape platform?

The scientists found that a ratio of 1 part omega-3 oils to every 4 parts omega-6 was ideal for rats. Rats on that diet consistently found the platform most rapidly and even returned to the site after the platform had been removed. Alter the ratio up or down, however, and learning ability declined. Interestingly, the scientists found that too much omega-3 (a ratio of 1 to 3) was just as damaging to the learning process as too little (a ratio of 1 to 6) in rats.

The Israeli team suggests that the results in rats might be extrapolated to humans. However, the unique structure and enormous energy requirements of the human brain set us apart. For humans, the questions of how much omega-6, how much omega-3, and which omega-3 depend in large part on the developmental age of the individual. For example, the fetus and newborn require large amounts of DHA and arachidonic acid, while older children and adults appear to require more EPA. In addition, the likelihood that someone on a Western diet might somehow consume too much omega-3 fatty acid is remote, provided the recommendations in this book are followed. Recall the traditional Inuit diet of 14 to 19 grams per day of omega-3, and the associated health benefits. On this point, a wide range of scientists agree. At a recent national meeting, leading nutritionists, paleoanthropologists, cardiologists, psychiatrists, and lipid chemists all concurred that, according to current data, the optimal dietary ratio of omega-6 to omega-3 fatty acids for humans should be approximately 1 to 1. Since omega-6 fatty acids are so abundant in our diet and omega-3s so scarce, it seems unlikely that anyone on the regimen suggested in this book could ever overdose on fish oil or other forms of omega-3 fatty acids. Nevertheless, we do recommend sticking to our guidelines or to those from other credible sources, and working with a healthcare provider if you are making large changes in your dietary intake of omega-3 fatty acids.

A definitive conclusion regarding omega-3 fatty acids and cognitive abilities in adults must await further research. Nonetheless, given that the omega-3s are remarkably safe and provide so many other benefits, choosing to supplement one's diet in the *hope* of a cognitive edge probably has no downside and may be the prudent thing to do.

12

Psychopharmacology and the Health Food Store

෴ The notion (correct or not) that we can avoid drugs and their negative side effects through the practice of natural, or alternative medicine (also known as complementary medicine)—herbs, acupuncture, hypnosis, and other popular remedies—has taken the West by storm. Bookstores devote entire sections to New Age healing. Television reporters relate the latest findings on non-Western cures. And most of us have either tried some form of alternative medicine ourselves or know someone who has turned to unconventional therapies—either in search of a more "natural" way to heal or when traditional treatments didn't work. More than a third of Americans are using some form of alternative medical care, spending an estimated $13.7 billion a year on such remedies, according to a recent article in the *New England Journal of Medicine*, by David Eisenberg, M.D., a Harvard physician studying alternative medicine practices.

Can they make us well? Often, yes. Although many healing methods do not live up to their claims or are untested, and some are harmful, several have earned the respect of mainstream med-

icine through research on their safety and efficacy. "As a physician," says Adriane Fugh-Berman, a medical officer at the National Institutes of Health and author of *Alternative Medicine:
What Works,* "I've seen scientific evidence of these therapies in
the form of clinical trials." Even so, it is a characteristic of many
alternative therapies that the actual mechanism of cure—the scientific explanation of how it affects the body—is often mysteri-
ous to a Westerner, because it is dependent on a different set of
scientific and philosophical assumptions, as, for example, the
"chi" or energy centers of Chinese medicine.

Omega-3 Fatty Acids and Complementary Medicine

Many people automatically think that anything "natural" be-
longs in the complementary medicine camp, and omega-3 fatty
acids have often been grouped in that category. Other natural
treatments for mood disorders, including St. John's wort and
SAMe (s-adenosylmethionine), have often been categorized as
complementary medicines as well, and not part of the allopathic
(conventional) medicine world.

Omega-3 essential fatty acids belong in both worlds. They are
natural; their path from phytoplankton to human beings is an elegant story of the natural world and the connections and inter-
dependence of different species. The understanding of this story
is also part of the world of Western science and medicine with its
focus on understanding the omega-3 molecules, the beauty of
their different chemical structures, and their interaction with
other molecules and systems in the body. As so eloquently stated
by Norman Salem, Jr., Ph.D., a leader in lipid biochemistry at
NIH and NIAAA, in reference to the importance of DHA in
brain and retinal development, "In fact, this may be the only case
in modern day biology where an alteration of the behavior of the
whole organism can be reasonably ascribed to a change in the
structure at the atomic level."

While omega-3 fatty acids are derived from natural marine or
terrestrial sources, from a Western medical standpoint, the
omega-3s have well-established biological effects, and their de-

pletion in Western societies is well documented. There are double-blind data showing their effectiveness and safety in treating a range of disorders, from cardiovascular disease and rheumatoid arthritis to Crohn's disease and bipolar disorder.

The fundamental difference between the omega-3s and both synthetic or herbal antidepressants is that the omega-3s are not used as an added, foreign substance to fix a problem. Supplying omega-3s appears to give back to the body what it requires and needs for proper functioning. The omega-3 fatty acids are essential building blocks of health that must be supplied in the diet—in food or supplement form. The ability of the omega-3s to improve so many conditions is a reflection of how depleted we are, and it emphasizes the disease states that have developed in response to a deficiency—possibly due to omega-3 stores depleted over several generations.

This ability to provide the body with what it needs to enhance health spans both complementary and Western medicine. Mainstream medicine is in the process of changing its focus on disease processes and is now beginning to focus also on the health of the whole person. Western medicine is opening up and learning about the many different ways of healing around the world and the different treatments used. Many substances found in nature can provide new and better ways of improving health and treating disease. Currently, researchers from many different fields are searching the earth for new biologically active plants before important sources of botanicals are destroyed. True to itself, Western medicine will continue to demand requirements of double-blind studies and scientifically valid research for efficacy and safety.

Complementary treatments are also coming to be known in the mainstream. The public is demanding that doctors pay attention to these natural or complementary treatments and learn to use them, or at least be aware of them. The public is also demanding that herbs and supplements be tested for their potency, purity, possible toxicities, and interactions with other treatments. People want to know whether the natural or complementary remedies are proven and safe. Sometimes such proof is hard to find. Within an herbal or natural remedy there may be more than one substance that is biologically active. In St. John's wort it is still unclear what molecular substance or combination of substances provides the mild mood-elevating action. Isolating the active compound(s) can be difficult. Western medicine has taken half a century to discover, separate, and begin to understand two crucial substances in fish oil, EPA and DHA.

Providing new hope by discovering new treatments, with an understanding of their molecular structure and the mechanisms of action in the body, has been one goal of my research. Helping people has been the other. The ideal medicine is that which without harm provides or brings the individual to as natural a state of good health as possible, regardless of the source of the treatment. We must ask that the world of different medicines come together with respect, each offering different but important ways to treat illness and increase health.

Are "Natural" Products Really Better?

Many people distinguish alternative medicine from Western medicine because of the use of natural products instead of synthetically manufactured medicines. Fundamentally, there is no

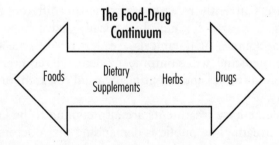

FIGURE 12–1: The Food-Drug Continuum

If something eaten influences the body, it is because of its biochemical action. Foods, supplements, herbs, and synthetic pharmaceuticals all affect the body in the same fundamental, chemical way. Omega-3 fatty acids can be considered food, a dietary supplement, or a drug, depending on your point of view.

difference between a synthetic and a natural version of a biologically derived compound if the molecular structures are identical. However, many biologically derived substances (i.e., substances obtained from plant or animal origins) can be very difficult to duplicate exactly. Often the naturally derived substance has a specific three-dimensional structure that is difficult to synthesize in the laboratory. This so-called stereochemistry is analogous to a plant producing a "left-handed" molecule while the synthetic version is a mixture of "left"- and "right"-handed molecules. Herbal treatments also often have more than one active principle, and possibly many different compounds in varying amounts required for biological activity, making the task of duplication more difficult.

Finally there is, for many reasons, an inherent appeal to using natural substances. For some it may be related to a spiritual or mystical reason, a belief that natural is better, a desire to be closer to nature or simpler times. For many people natural substances simply feel less like being on a drug and are more acceptable.

Some extremists, however, believe that "natural" is automatically safer and more desirable than a synthetic pharmaceutical product. But even the identification of what is "natural" can be confusing. For example, lithium is one of the few FDA-approved "drugs" for bipolar disorder. Lithium is seen by some as a toxic drug representing the establishment in psychiatry. Yet it is an element found in the periodic chart—in other words, as simple a natural substance as can be. Conversely, many natural substances are highly toxic: cyanide, strychnine, curare, and arsenic, for example. In addition, with the lack of regulatory supervision of manufacturing processes, what goes into an herbal or dietary supplement may be suspect.

Both conventional Western medicine and many forms of alternative and complementary medicine have much to offer humanity in reducing suffering and improving health. Integrating different medical philosophies and practices can be difficult, but it is well worth the effort.

In natural, herbal, and complementary, as well as in conventional Western medical treatments, evaluation of the substance for efficacy, safety, side effects, purity, quality, interactions with other medicines taken, and how it works in the body will always be important.

With this in mind, it is easy to see why the omega-3 fatty acids are claimed by both traditional physicians and advocates of complementary medicine.

Complementary Medicine in Mood Disorders: A Primer for Understanding the Use of St. John's Wort and SAMe

St. John's wort and SAMe are two of the most commonly used complementary treatments for mood disorders, primarily unipolar major depression. In my psychiatric practice, I try to combine the allopathic (traditional-conventional psychopharmacology with or without psychotherapy) and complementary medicine treatments when they seem appropriate. Other complementary remedies used to treat depression or bipolar disorder can be divided into two major categories: symptom control (for example, St. John's wort to treat depressive symptoms) and side-effect control (for example, gingerroot to treat nausea associated with certain medications). Appendix A has more information regarding complementary medicine therapies in psychiatry.

Anyone who intends to try St. John's wort, SAMe, or any other substance for depression should do so only under medical supervision. Self-treatment of depression is potentially dangerous. If you think you might be depressed, you should consult your health-care professional. This section will provide information for those interested in understanding these supplements and how they are used.

St. John's Wort (Hypericum perforatum)

History. St. John's wort has been used for millennia to treat a variety of disorders. The word *hypericum* is an ancient Greek word (*hyper* = "above" and *icum* = "icon") translated roughly as "above spirits," hinting at how long physicians have known about the mood effects of this widespread herb. St. John's wort has also been used as a topical antiseptic for wounds. The name St. John's wort derives from the blood-red berries (resembling stigmata) the plant produces, but *also* because folklore says that the flowers bloom on St. John's Day (June 24).

Strength of Data Supporting Antidepressant Action. There are more than twenty controlled studies of St. John's wort in major depression, almost all from Germany. Taken together, the data are sufficiently strong to conclude that St. John's wort is very likely an effective antidepressant. However, there are major and minor flaws in the design of every one of these published studies. For example, all of the studies examined individuals with mild to moderate depression; no study treated patients with severe or treatment-resistant major depression. Another problem is that many of the studies were comparative trials—comparing St. John's wort to an existing antidepressant. There are two problems with this approach. First, none of the comparative studies used the SSRI (selective serotonin reuptake inhibitors) class of antidepressants. The SSRIs, the prototype of which is Prozac, are now the standard antidepressant drugs around the world. Thus, there are no data to indicate whether the antidepressant effects of St. John's wort are inferior, superior, or equivalent to the SSRIs.

The second problem with comparative studies is the lack of a placebo control. Placebos are inactive substances matched to look just like the real medication. Double-blind, placebo-controlled clinical trials remain the only way to be sure a treatment has true biological activity. This is especially important in research involving people with only mild to moderate depressive symptoms, because placebo response rates in these individuals range from 30 to 40 percent.

To settle the issue once and for all, the National Institutes of Health has recently funded the largest and best designed St. John's wort trial to date. This study will be a coordinated effort of several research centers and will compare three different experimental groups. A standardized and accepted form of St. John's wort will be compared to Zoloft (an SSRI) and also to a placebo. The hope is that this study will definitively clarify the antidepressant effects of St. John's wort.

Possible Benefits over Conventional Antidepressant Medications. If it is truly effective in major depression, St. John's wort would be most useful in those with mild to moderate depressive symptoms. There is little or no evidence that St. John's wort is effective in severe depression or in those with major depression who have not responded to standard trials of antidepressants. The short-term side-effect profile of St. John's is only slightly better than some of the newer conventional antidepressants, such as the SSRIs (Prozac, Zoloft, Paxil, Luvox, and Celexa), Effexor XR, and Wellbutrin SR. However, St. John's wort does not produce two crucial, long-term side effects of the SSRIs and Effexor XR: inhibited sexual functioning (loss of sex drive and delayed or diminished orgasm) and potential weight gain. Sexual side effects and weight gain also do not occur with some conventional antidepressants, such as Serzone and Wellbutrin SR.

Another possible advantage of St. John's wort is the long history of use as a traditional herbal medicine. Although this long experience has failed to document any severe toxicity, it would be desirable to have formal toxicity studies, such as the tests the FDA requires for prescription medication. Some people reject the notion of conventional pharmaceutical treatment for many disorders, including major depression. For these individuals, St. John's wort and the other so-called natural mood-elevating agents are a useful option when closely monitored.

Drawbacks. There are several drawbacks to the use of St. John's wort:

- Toxicity. St. John's wort is a relatively benign substance when used as directed. If side effects do occur, they tend to be mild. However, because of its antidepressant activity, there is a risk of inducing mania or increasing the frequency of mood swings in patients with bipolar disorder. This so-called switch process may be a bigger problem than it seems because many of those with mild to moderate forms of bipolar disorder are in the community and are unaware they even have this disorder. They may self-medicate manic or irritable states with alcohol or other substances. When depressed, these individuals may try an herbal mood-elevating substance such as St. John's wort. Extrapolating from what is known about the switch process with conventional antidepressants, approximately 20 to 50 percent of those with bipolar disorder may be at risk for manic switch when receiving St. John's wort over the long term.

- Self-treatment of depression. Although St. John's wort has little danger associated with its pharmacological activity, one distinct hazard is the risk of self-treatment of major depression. This is dangerous because major depression is a potentially lethal condition due to the risk of suicide. Self-treatment of major depression with suicidal features is a hazardous undertaking. Part of the danger stems from the observation that in some depressed patients who are actually responding to an antidepressant, the early period of recovery is the most dangerous time. This is because increased energy may precede improved mood and heighten the depressed individual's capacity to carry out a suicidal impulse. The message with St. John's wort or any other complementary medicine treatment for anything but the mildest form of major depression is that people should not self-medicate and should be closely monitored by trained mental health professionals.
- Drug interaction risks. St. John's wort has effects on the neurotransmitter serotonin. Mixing St. John's wort with other antidepressants (many of which also have serotonergic activity) can lead to a dangerous overactivity of serotonin systems in the body and brain, known as "serotonin syndrome."
- Common side effects. Nausea, agitation, increased sunburn risk.
- Rare side effects. Induction of mania, insomnia, serotonin syndrome.

- Lack of external quality control and limited data on safety and effectiveness. St. John's wort has one major drawback it shares with all so-called dietary supplements. In 1994, the U.S. Congress, under intense lobbying pressure, passed the Dietary Supplements, Health, and Education Act, sponsored by Senator Orrin Hatch (R-Utah), which stripped the FDA of its authority to regulate dietary supplements. Thus, we must trust the manufacturer and package labels regarding the contents of their products.

We will likely never see safety and effectiveness studies of the quality and magnitude of those done for conventional pharmaceutical products. Like other herbal treatments, St. John's wort is of little interest to mainstream pharmaceutical companies because patents are by and large unobtainable. Without the support of industry, completing these prohibitively expensive, large-scale studies is exceedingly difficult, if not impossible.

How Supplied. St. John's wort is supplied in several forms:

- *Capsules.* This is the most popular form of St. John's wort, because it is convenient, standardized, readily available, and familiar to Americans. The most common form of capsule uses a standardized extract of St. John's wort containing 0.3 percent hypericin. Hypericin is a chemical found in the St. John's wort plant, but it does not have antidepressant activity. The active antidepressant compound or compounds for St. John's wort remain unknown. However, whatever the active compound or compounds are, they are present in standardized extracts of hypericin. Probably the biggest advantage of using capsules containing the standardized 0.3 percent extract of hypericin is that many of the clinical trials of St. John's wort have used this formulation. This provides some degree of certainty that the capsule contains a known and reasonably proven effective formulation. The designation LI 160 indicates a very high-quality form of the 0.3 percent hypericin extract used in research studies.
- *Elixirs.* Some experienced practitioners recommend elixirs

containing standard alcohol extracts of St. John's wort. These are prepared by mixing the ground plant material with warm ethanol (ethyl alcohol). The alcohol extract is then filtered to remove the residual plant material and stored in opaque bottles until used.

- *Other forms.* Many health-food stores have numerous St. John's wort preparations on their shelves. These include the raw plant material, tea bags, and combination products containing other herbal medications along with the St. John's wort. Anyone who begins therapy with one of these less standardized preparations and does not respond will not know whether his or her depression does not respond to St. John's wort or if the preparation used was inadequate.

Standard Usage. Generally it is used as follows: as capsules of St. John's wort standardized extract, each containing 300 milligrams 0.3 percent hypericin. The starting dosage is one 300-milligram capsule by mouth twice per day (morning and night). After three to four days, if there are no side effects, the dosage can be increased to two capsules each morning and one capsule at night (some practitioners prefer to divide the dosage further and give 300 milligrams three times per day). This total daily dosage of 900 milligrams of 0.3 percent hypericin extract is an adequate dosage for many people.

The antidepressant effects of St. John's wort may be delayed by two to six weeks. If there is no response by week two or three, the dosage may be increased to two capsules (600 milligrams) twice per day. The maximum recommended dosage is approximately 900 milligrams per day, but extreme dosages of 1,200 to 1,500 milligrams per day have been used under certain circumstances.

SAMe (S-Adenosylmethionine)

History. SAMe has received recent publicity as an effective and "natural" antidepressant with few, if any, side effects: the reason for the recent media attention is unclear, since SAMe has been studied intermittently as an antidepressant for nearly thirty years. The use of SAMe as an antidepressant was originally motivated by discoveries in the 1960s and 1970s regarding SAMe and the biochemical processes regulating the activity of norepinephrine and serotonin, two neurotransmitters that were just being recognized for their role in the development of major depression.

SAMe is found naturally in the body and the brain. It is not an essential nutrient because the human body does synthesize SAMe from readily available precursors. Some researchers have speculated that SAMe can be depleted if there is a deficiency in certain other nutrients, such as the amino acid methionine (the immediate precursor to SAMe) and vitamins B_{12} and folic acid. However, the medical literature contains contradictory reports regarding whether SAMe is depleted in psychiatric disorders. Nonetheless, SAMe has an important function in the structure of phospholipids located in the cell membrane, perhaps altering their function in cell signaling. Precisely how this signaling is involved in mood regulation is unknown, but there appears to be a connection between membrane phospholipid structure, cell signaling, and mood.

Strength of Data Supporting Antidepressant Action. There have been dozens of scientific papers published over the past thirty years regarding the effects of SAMe in those with psychiatric disorders. Most claims regarding the antidepressant effects of SAMe stem from research on intravenous SAMe in major depression, where SAMe is injected directly into a vein. A recent media account reported that more than forty "clinical studies" of SAMe in approximately fourteen hundred patients have been published. However, a computer search (via Medline) of the medical literature revealed only about fifteen actual clinical trials of SAMe in depression. Many of these studies were performed in Italy, and the majority were open-label clinical trials of oral SAMe. "Open-label" means that the patients and researchers knew that SAMe was being administered. Open-label studies are crucial (this is where most medical discoveries are made), but they are also associated with the placebo effect and falsely high response rates often occur.

Among the handful of controlled trials of SAMe in major depression, the strongest findings are associated with the intravenous route of administration rather than the oral one.

Notwithstanding the limitations of the scientific studies, a critical review of the literature indicates that SAMe is likely to be an effective antidepressant. More research is required to define response rates and develop clinical or biochemical predictors of SAMe response.

Possible Benefits of SAMe over Conventional Antidepressant Medications. There are virtually no side effects associated with SAMe in depressed patients correctly diagnosed with unipolar depression.

Although SAMe is generally contraindicated for individuals with bipolar disorder because it has a high potential to provoke a rapid switch into mania, it might be considered if other treatment options have been unsuccessful. Because it activates the switch process to the dangerous, manic phase of the disorder, those with bipolar disorder should consider SAMe only under the supervision of a psychiatrist experienced in psychiatric medication.

Drawbacks. There are several drawbacks to the use of SAMe:

* Induces mania in bipolar patients at an extremely high rate. While at least one in ten people with depression in the general population suffer from bipolar disorder, that rate increases to more than one in four for depressed individuals who seek treatment. Many of these people have a hidden bipolar disorder, either waiting to emerge or previously unrecognized and undiagnosed. Thus, without careful screening for a history of bipolar symptoms, many cases of mania associated with the use of SAMe can be expected. While all antidepressants can induce mania in susceptible patients,

SAMe appears to induce mania more rapidly and at a much higher frequency than conventional prescription antidepressants. For example, less than 25 percent of bipolar patients receiving an SSRI, such as Prozac, without a concomitant mood stabilizer can be expected to switch into mania over a one-year period. For SAMe, the rate of mania induction may be as high as 50 percent within two to three weeks.

SAMe should be considered for use with bipolar type I individuals only when a number of other treatments have failed, and only then under supervision by an experienced clinician. SAMe would be somewhat safer in patients with bipolar disorder type II, characterized by a mild form of pathological mood elevation along with severe, often chronic depression. SAMe should be avoided for any bipolar patient who has experienced rapid-cycling symptoms, defined as four or more separate mood episodes in the previous twelve months.

- Instability. Due to the chemical instability of the compound and the unregulated nature of the dietary supplement industry, concern over the integrity, stability, and potency of SAMe preparations persists.
- Additional studies validating the antidepressant value of oral SAMe must still be done.
- High cost. Because the therapeutic oral dosage may be as high as 1,600 milligrams per day, the monthly cost of SAMe may exceed $360. This is prohibitively high for most patients.
- Limited data on safety and effectiveness. Like St. John's wort, SAMe has never undergone the rigorous safety testing required for prescription medications. Although the existing data suggest that SAMe appears safe in short-term trials, no long-term data exist. One possible complication of long-term SAMe use is increased risk of heart attack as it appears to increase the serum concentration of homocysteine, a known risk factor in heart disease. Further studies need to be done.

How supplied. SAMe is supplied in 200-milligram coated tablets.

Standard Usage. Starting dosage is 200 milligrams by mouth twice per day, increased every two to three days until a dosage of 400 milligrams to 800 milligrams twice per day is achieved. The usual maximum dosage is 1,600 milligrams per day, divided into two or three parts.

The use of SAMe is fairly straightforward. In mild unipolar major depression, it may be used if the clinician and patient choose this agent over conventional prescription antidepressants or other natural mood-elevating substances, such as St. John's wort or omega-3 fatty acids. In moderate or severe depression, especially where suicidal thoughts or safety is an issue, SAMe should be used only as an adjunct to more standard prescription antidepressant therapies.

SAMe is generally not to be used in those with a suspected diagnosis of bipolar disorder. It should also be avoided in depressed individuals under age twenty-five who are at high risk of developing bipolar disorder in the future.

Part II

THE OMEGA-3 RENEWAL PLAN

13

The Omega-3 Renewal Plan: Optimizing Your Mood and Health with Omega-3 Essential Fatty Acids

☙ Western medicine is only now discovering what many non-Western cultures have long known: that a balance of forces is crucial to health. In addition, Western medicine is realizing that we really are what we eat. There is a direct relationship between the composition of our food and the composition of our body. Among other things, the amount and ratio of omega-6 to omega-3, which affects our mood and health, depends solely on diet.

Creating a New Paradigm of Health

Understanding the elegant and biologically powerful balance between omega-6 and omega-3 fatty acids is creating a new paradigm of health. An altered and hostile internal chemistry is created by an imbalance in the dietary ratio of omega-6 to omega-3. Excess omega-6 fatty acids cause an increase in the production of certain cell-signaling molecules, such as the cytokine inter-leukin-1 and the eicosanoid molecules prostaglandin E2 and leukotriene B4. These omega-6–derived molecules appear to promote depression, inflammation, excess blood clotting, and constriction of the arteries. These molecules can act directly on neurons, affecting neurotransmitter levels and receptors—actions that regulate mood. Small amounts of the omega-6, arachidonic acid, are necessary and healthy for neurons, and they promote growth. But too much arachidonic acid is toxic to neurons and can even cause cell damage or death. By increasing the amount of EPA and omega-3–derived eicosanoids, we counteract the toxic, depressive, and disease-promoting actions of excess omega-6 and create a healthier, more balanced state.

Increasing the omega-3s in our diet also provides cells with the proper balance of lipids (fats) needed for the fluidity of the cell membrane. The omega-3 fatty acids DHA and EPA increase the mobility and fluidity of cell membranes. Proper membrane fluidity permits receptors, ion channels, and other cell-signaling molecules in the membrane to function normally, which is also important for mood regulation.

Not knowing about the omega-3 deficiency that our culture has developed, we have come to accept as natural the widespread occurrence of diseases such as depression (for which we have long blamed ourselves or our parents), heart disease, rheumatoid arthritis, and diabetes. But we can now see how our deficiency in omega-3s places us at risk for these modern illnesses. Our current ratio of omega-6 and omega-3 is far from the Paleolithic ideal ratio of one to one. In the United States, we eat up to twenty times more omega-6 than omega-3. This high ratio can dramatically disrupt our biochemistry, affecting our moods, our ability to handle the growing stress of everyday life, and the health of virtually every system of our bodies. Lacking sufficient omega-3 stores, our bodies remain in a constant state of stress and distress, with hormones and other chemical messengers spinning out of control, causing or worsening many of today's health problems.

Knowledge is power, so set your goals and get ready for change. The Omega-3 Renewal Plan provides healthful and practical ways to replenish your body with omega-3 fatty acids, redesign your diet and lifestyle, and move step by step toward boosting your overall mental and physical health.

The beneficial changes acquired from replenishing the body's stores of omega-3 fatty acids may take from several weeks to several months to occur. However, some individuals may begin to feel the positive effects as quickly as two to four days after beginning omega-3 supplements. For some, changes in mood and health may take longer. Be patient, and know that you are making powerful and restorative changes in your body's biology, in your ability to feel good and handle stress, and in your resistance to the diseases of modern times.

The Scientific Basis of the Omega-3 Connection

The Omega-3 Renewal Plan is a clear, stepwise program for restoring the omega-3 essential fatty acids your body needs for well-being and health. The program is based on hundreds of scientific studies showing the benefits of omega-3s to human health. This scientific evidence is the foundation of the Omega-3 Renewal Plan.

Omega-3 essential fatty acids must be obtained from diet since the human body cannot synthesize them. Scientific studies of modern populations that have escaped many of the diseases of the West, such as the Inuit and other traditional populations still consuming high omega-3 diets, provide a model of past human omega-3 consumption. The amount of omega-3 that these cultures traditionally ingest on a daily basis is huge and can act as a guide for setting our maximum daily intake. The Inuit have few dietary options due to their limiting environment and may consume up to 19 grams of omega-3 per day.

Given the safety of omega-3s and the numerous health benefits they provide, I feel comfortable recommending omega-3 fatty acids for my patients, my friends, and my family. Of course each individual's health and biology are unique. It is essential that you consult with your own health-care provider prior to implementing any significant change in your diet or beginning dietary supplements. Although further research is needed and is ongoing, the Omega-3 Renewal Plan provides a starting point, combining our current omega-3 knowledge with other known health-enhancing techniques to improve mood, emotional well-being, and overall health.

The Paleolithic Diet: Stone Age Food in the Twenty-First Century

Our bodies and minds function and feel best when we respect our evolutionary biology. We were meant to eat a diet high in green leafy vegetables, fruits, fish, nuts, lean protein from wild game, and carbohydrates and fiber from vegetables, tubers, and fruits. Humans did not evolve eating large amounts of grains, processed carbohydrates, refined sugars, fats, or oils. In returning to the diet of our down-to-earth ancestors, we give our bodies the best chance for health. We also give ourselves the opportunity to help or prevent depression, heart disease, diabetes, inflammatory disorders, and other modern ailments.

A Paleolithic diet incorporates lots of colorful fruits, green leafy vegetables, fish, beans and other legumes, lean meat, nuts, and some carbohydrates from whole grains, root and tuber vegetables, and bread. Many of these foods contain powerful phytonutrients, such as bioflavonoids, which include powerful antioxidants and many other substances that are health enhancing. Plant-based, fiber-rich foods should be consumed in high amounts. Many herbs and spices also contain potent antioxidants and are beneficial.

Increase Fruits and Vegetables and Omega-3s

The Paleolithic diet is very similar to both the modern Mediterranean diet and the plant-based diet. However, the Mediterranean diet has slightly more breads and greater reliance on grains. Another dietary guide, the "food pyramid," has been criticized for recommending too few servings of fruits and vegetables and too many servings of simple and complex carbohydrates. The Omega-3 Renewal Plan uses elements from these, and other nutritional systems, as well as incorporating new research data on nutrition and essential fatty acids. I recommend increasing fruits and vegetables to five to seven servings per day and decreasing all fats except omega-3s.

Eat Whole Foods

It is probably best to eat nutrient-rich whole foods: whole foods are unprocessed, and they may contain many nutrients and phytochemicals that cannot be obtained in supplements. Positive synergistic reactions between different phytochemicals in plants may be lost when they are not eaten in plant form. Try to buy or even grow organic foods and naturally raised animal products. Many pesticides are potent and damaging chemicals whose capacity to cause neurological disorders as well as cancer, allergies and hypersensitivity reactions remains under-studied.

Antioxidant Facts

Antioxidants are mentioned frequently in the nutrition and supplement literature. Antioxidants are important because oxidative damage caused by free radicals can damage omega-3 or omega-6 fatty acids in the membrane, as well as harm other crucial biochemicals, such as DNA. Free radicals are molecules that have an unpaired electron. They are highly chemically reactive and will pull an electron off other molecules, leaving the other molecule damaged or oxidized. Once the molecule is oxidized, it may lose its function and may also oxidize other surrounding molecules. Cell membranes are vulnerable to oxidative damage. Omega-3 and omega-6 essential fatty acids are vulnerable, due to the so-called cis ("on the same side") configuration of their double bonds. Unhealthy trans-fatty acids have a different configuration of double bonds, which makes them much more resistant to oxidation, but they have been unequivocally shown to be unhealthful for the body.

Dietary Recommendations

Three basic classes of biochemicals comprise food: protein, carbohydrates, and fat.

Protein. We do not require the large amounts of protein most Americans eat. I recommend eating four ounces daily of fish, lean meat, eggs, beans, or other legumes for protein. Try to eat some protein with each meal. If you are a vegetarian, it is important that your food include the essential amino acids, which are the basic building blocks of proteins. It is often difficult for vegans (strict vegetarians) to obtain some essential amino acids, commonly found in animal products.

Fish is a good protein source, because it is low in saturated fat. Two to three servings of ocean water fish per week may be healthful. However, it is important to be aware of where the fish was caught and make informed decisions regarding contaminants. Freshwater fish from lakes or rivers that have been contaminated can contain large amounts of heavy metals and carcinogens—especially fish that feed on the lake floor, where the contaminated sludge settles. Also, you need to be aware that if the fish is farm raised, it may have been fed terrestrial food devoid of omega-3s and therefore contain little or no omega-3s in its body. Oily ocean fish contain the most omega-3s. The omega-3s are concentrated in the dark muscle, where it provides the fish with a near-perfect form of energy for long ocean migration.

For meat dishes, you are better off with free-range animals that have grazed on wild plants. This meat contains more of the short-chain omega-3 ALA versus the high omega-6 in grain-fed animals. Free-range chickens and their eggs are good sources of protein and also provide a small amount of omega-3s. Commercial eggs from chickens, which are fed fishmeal, are now available and some brands contain very high amounts of EPA and DHA. Dairy sources of protein are fine and can be used if the amount of fat is kept low.

Egg yolks, long banished from the breakfast table, are extremely good for you. The yolk naturally contains lutein and zeaxanthin, which are light-absorbing biochemical pigments that are powerful antioxidants. A recent study suggests they may protect the lens of the eye from cataract formation due to oxidative damage by ultraviolet radiation. Lecithin, another component of egg yolk, is an important constituent of all cell membranes. If you limit yourself to one egg per day, the cholesterol content should not be excessive.

Nuts in small quantities are excellent sources of protein and oleic acid. Oleic acid is a monounsaturated fatty acid that appears to protect LDLs and membranes from oxidation. Nuts also contain nutrients such as zinc, magnesium, and potassium. Pecans and walnuts also contain the omega-3 ALA.

The family of plant foods known as legumes includes peas, soybeans, and various other beans, and all are good sources of protein. Soybeans contain the antioxidant, cancer-fighting isoflavones genistein and daidzein.

Carbohydrates. Root vegetables, like turnips and carrots, and tubers, such as sweet potatoes and yams, are more nutritious sources of carbohydrates than grains. All are rich in vitamins, minerals, fiber, and bioflavonoids. Limit the amount of carbohydrates from cereals and processed flour, and cut out high-carbohydrate, high-fat foods such as potato chips, French fries, and other fast foods. Use whole grains and whole grain bread, but limit the servings to three or less per day.

Most people do not realize that the antioxidants contained in fruits and vegetables only last 4 to 6 hours in the body. For this reason, one should aim for seven servings of fruits and vegetables each day. Leafy and cruciferous vegetables such as broccoli are excellent sources of vitamins, minerals, and fiber. Dark-green leafy vegetables such as kale, spinach, parsley, and cruciferous vegetables contain coenzyme Q10 and glutathione, both components of cell-protecting antioxidant systems. Richly pigmented fruits and vegetables such as blueberries, cantaloupe, watermelon, and red peppers also provide antioxidant phytochemicals. Tomatoes contain both alpha- and beta-carotene, as well as lycopene, an extremely powerful antioxidant. Even the green herbs rosemary, oregano, and thyme have antioxidant compounds.

Substitute these healthy foods for the processed commercial snacks high in carbohydrates and trans-fatty acids that are so common today. Cut the fruits and vegetables up ahead of time, if possible, so you have something easy to reach for.

Fats and Oils. It is essential to cut down on all fats and oils except omega-3 oils, which you are increasing. For cooking oils, use olive or canola. Both are primarily made of monounsaturated fats. Olive oil contains the most oleic acid, a monounsaturated fat, which is an important component of cell membranes. In the membrane, oleic acid has antioxidant qualities, which protect other fatty acids, including omega-3s, from oxidation.

The best olive oil is virgin or extra virgin olive oil, made from the first pressings of the olives, and is the least oxidized. Olive oil also has phytochemicals that may be beneficial. Buy olive oil in small quantities in opaque containers, because it oxidizes easily when exposed to light and air. Olive oil also contains some omega-6 oils, a smaller amount of omega-3, and some saturated fat.

Canola oil is composed primarily of the monounsaturated erucic acid made from rapeseeds. Among oils it contains the least amount of saturated fat. It is less expensive than olive oil and has a less distinct flavor, which some prefer. Be careful not to purchase hydrogenated or heat-stabilized oils which contain unhealthy amounts of trans-fatty acids. Extra oleic safflower or extra oleic sunflower oil is also good. Avoid regular sunflower oil, safflower oil, and corn oil due to their high omega-6 content. In small quantities, butter is less harmful than the trans-fatty acids found in margarine. However, all oils and fats compete for inclusion in the membrane and for receptor sites, and so it is important to reduce consumption of all non-omega-3 fats.

Commercial snacks contain many unhealthy fats, including saturated fat, trans-fatty acids, and omega-6 fatty acids. Omega-6 fats, so prevalent in seed oils, directly compete with omega-3s. You need to reduce your intake of omega-6 whenever possible to work toward the ideal one-to-one ratio of omega-6 to omega-3.

Some people worry about not getting enough omega-6. But our diet is so skewed toward omega-6 that there is little worry. A Stone Age or Mediterranean diet, with fish and olive oil, will provide you with ample omega-6.

Why Not Just Eat More Fish?

The Omega-3 Renewal Plan includes high-quality omega-3 supplements if necessary along with a moderate intake of fish and specific plants as sources of omega-3 fatty acids. It would be very difficult, and possibly dangerous, to try to get high amounts of omega-3 fatty acids from eating just fish. It would take somewhere between 6 and 32 typical cans of tuna per day to achieve the omega-3 dosage we used in our bipolar study. (Different tuna species have differing amounts of omega-3 in their bodies.) Old and new peer-reviewed research studies documenting the potential dangers of fish consumption due to contamination with heavy metals (such as mercury) or organochlorine carcinogens (cancer-causing pollutants such as PCBs) should make anyone pause before eating large amounts of certain fish. Corroborating the research are alarming reports from government agencies regarding the dangers of excessive fish consumption.

The Web site of the Vermont State Board of Health suggests that more than even one can of tuna per week delivers too much toxic mercury to adults. Children are at even higher risk because of their smaller body size, as well as the increased vulnerability of a developing nervous system to the toxic effects of mercury.

The FDA's Web site lists extensive information on fish contamination around the world. In general, freshwater fish in the United States and many other regions of the world are more likely to be contaminated than ocean species of fish.

The FDA takes no official position on ocean species of fish. Ocean fish, such as salmon, mackerel, and some other types of oily fish, can deliver more omega-3 per serving than most other fish species. These fish store the omega-3 fatty acids in their flesh (muscles), while non-oily, "white" fish species (such as cod) store the omega-3 fatty acids in their livers. The degree of contamination among fish species that are living in the open ocean is unclear. The South Polar region is less polluted than oceans in the Northern Hemisphere. In addition, large predatory fish with long life spans will accumulate toxins in their fatty tissues, while smaller fish species, which are lower on the food chain and have relatively shorter life spans (such as anchovies, sardines, and menhaden), will be far less contaminated.

One way to decrease toxins in fish is to farm them. In fact, the majority of salmon eaten in developed countries is farm-raised. Farm-raised fish have the obvious advantage of being less prone to contamination from toxins in the open ocean. However, recall that fish cannot make omega-3 fatty acids themselves; they depend on their food to supply these essential oils. In Western Europe, salmon farmers are usually careful to feed the fish with products from the ocean, which contain high amounts of omega-3 fatty acids. In the United States, some fish farms feed the salmon, at least partially, with land-based food, which has little or no omega-3 fatty acids. Thus, some U.S. farm-raised salmon may have less omega-3 fatty acids in their bodies, essentially reducing the key element making oily fish uniquely healthy. There is no easy way to determine what food was used in raising the fish purchased in a store or restaurant. Perhaps in the future, labels on fish will include omega-3 fatty acid content and results of testing for toxins.

14

Understanding Omega-3 Supplements

 Diet is essential. The core of the Omega-3 Renewal Plan is increased consumption of omega-3–rich foods and the use of omega-3 fatty acid supplements from two main sources: fish oils and flaxseed oil.

Fish Oil

Most of the clinical data on omega-3 fatty acids involves fish oil and its omega-3 components. Fish oil contains the two primary long-chain omega-3 fatty acids, EPA and DHA (see Chapter 2). DHA is generally incorporated into the cell membranes found throughout the body, but it is found in highest concentration in the retina, brain, and sperm. DHA is crucial for normal brain development and optimal cognitive and visual functioning in the fetus and newborn. The body holds on tightly to DHA; even moderate amounts of DHA in the diet (100–200 milligrams per day of DHA for an adult) appear adequate to sustain healthy levels. However, pregnant and nursing women have higher requirements due to the demands of the fetus and newborn for large quantities of omega-3s. A recent international conference sponsored by NIH recommended at least 300 milligrams per day of DHA for a pregnant or lactating woman.

EPA is the active anti-inflammatory omega-3. In health, the body should be in a non-inflammatory state, achieved by having sufficent quantities of EPA to keep the pro-inflammatory omega-6 arachidonic acid in check. Current evidence is pointing toward EPA as the most mood-promoting agent in fish oil, although further research may show that DHA is important as well. However, there is anecdotal data suggesting that too much DHA relative to EPA may cause a worsening of mood. I therefore recommend using a supplement with as high an EPA content as possible. More systematic studies are required to verify this clinical observation. There are now supplements available with EPA-to-DHA ratios of two-to-one all the way up to seven-to-one.

EPA is generally found in nearly twice the concentration of DHA in commonly available over-the-counter fish oil supplements. It is incorporated to a far lesser degree into cell membrane lipids when compared with DHA. However, even this relatively small amount of EPA incorporated into the membrane is extremely important and has strong biological activity in a number of processes in the brain and body. For example, EPA released from the membrane has powerful anti-inflammatory and ion-channel-modulating actions.

The turnover rate of EPA is high, so it must be replenished daily through the diet for optimal function. Besides its action from the membrane, EPA is also active as it circulates in the bloodstream, competing with its omega-6 fatty acid counterpart arachidonic acid in numerous biochemical pathways involving the eicosanoids. Once again, it is this balance between omega-3 fatty acids and omega-6 fatty acids that may be crucial to the observed clinical effects of EPA.

Dosage

If you are using the omega-3 fatty acids for health, mood, or cognitive enhancement, 1 to 2 grams (1000-2000 milligrams) daily of total omega-3 fatty acids (EPA plus DHA) is probably adequate. If you are using them for mood elevation or stabilization, a higher amount is sometimes required. Our bipolar disorder study, described in Chapter 7, used 9.6 grams of omega-3 fatty acids per day (6.2 grams EPA and 3.4 grams DHA). Clinically, usually 2 to 5 grams of omega-3 per day is adequate.

With the emerging data on EPA, I have begun to use the EPA content alone to calculate dosage requirements. Generally 1.5 to 4 grams per day of EPA is adequate to improve mood in patients with mood disorders. I have no experience using EPA in dosages exceeding 8 grams per day, but higher levels seem to be safe, since the traditional Greenland Eskimo diet consisted of up to 14 grams per day.

Anyone taking an anticlotting agent such as warfarin (Coumadin), or high doses of aspirin and related drugs, should talk to their health-care provider before taking omega-3 and vitamin E so they can be monitored for safety. In addition, anti-obesity medications that block the absorption of fats, such as Xenical, can also interfere with omega-3 absorption.

Under no circumstances should you lower or discontinue your medication by yourself. In some cases, individuals, working closely with their clinicians, have been able to lower the dosage of their medication. Also, although omega-3 is essential during pregnancy, I strongly recommend that women work with their health-care provider on using the supplements.

If your health-care provider is unfamiliar with the importance of omega-3 and its benefits, you can help to educate him or her and thus benefit others.

Using the Omega-3 Renewal Plan in Depression and Bipolar Disorder

In cases of moderate or severe depressive symptoms, the Omega-3 Renewal Plan is usually only used in addition to conventional psychopharmacological treatment. In certain individuals with only mild mood symptoms (for both depression and certain mild forms of bipolar disorder), I have used the plan alone, instead of conventional medication. This is justified as long as the patient's safety and well-being are not compromised. The advantage of using the plan first, instead of conventional mood drugs, lies in its safety and excellent side-effect profile. If increasing the amount of omega-3 fatty acids and implementing the other elements of the Omega-3 Renewal Plan fail to relieve mood symptoms, conventional medications (antidepressants and/or mood stabilizers) can then be tried.

I have also treated individuals who have moderate or severe mood symptoms with the Omega-3 Renewal Plan when conventional medications were not an option. For example, some individuals will not use conventional medications based on their religious or philosophical beliefs. Others have not responded to even multiple trials of conventional drugs, and some patients cannot tolerate standard mood drugs due to severe side effects. In these cases, it may be justified to use the Omega-3 Renewal Plan alone. However, in my practice, I have observed that conventional medications are sometimes more useful following the implementation of the Omega-3 Renewal Plan. This may be because some previously difficult-to-treat patients respond favorably to conventional medications once their brain is provided with an adequate amount of omega-3 fatty acids to function and respond normally. This restoration of response to conventional medication can occur even if the omega-3 fatty acids themselves do not seem to be reducing the mood symptoms. This clinical observation of restoration of response requires scientific confirmation.

Another favorable aspect of the omega-3 fatty acids is their compatibility with the whole range of psychiatric medications, other prescription and non-prescription medication, and most herbal treatments. The omega-3 fatty acids can be safely mixed with whatever medication you may be currently receiving. The only known exceptions may be blood thinners, such as high-dose aspirin (or similar drugs, such as ibuprofen) or warfarin (Coumadin). Because the omega-3 fatty acids tend to inhibit platelet action, combining the omega-3 fatty acids with a medication that may promote abnormal bleeding may increase the risk of bleeding even further. However, no case of such an interaction has ever been reported, and the danger of bleeding from an interaction between the omega-3s and a blood thinner would likely be extremely small with ordinary dosages of fish oil and blood thinners. A recent study confirmed this by demonstrating that low-dose aspirin used to prevent heart attack posed no hazard to someone receiving even large dosages of omega-3 fatty acids. Individual responses can vary. There have been reported cases of hypomania and mania, particularly with flaxseed oil (ALA). It is unclear if these reactions were due to the flaxseed oil or were part of that person's pattern of mood cycling. Either way, close monitoring of mood and health is indicated. You should never self-treat depression or bipolar disorder. Work with your health-care provider.

Choosing a Fish Oil Supplement

There are literally dozens of omega-3 dietary supplements available in health-food stores, pharmacies, Web sites, and catalogs. Omega-3 supplements are available in a variety of concentrations and characteristics. These supplements range from the highest pharmaceutical quality formulations to products of poor quality containing oxidized fish oil and possibly other contaminants.

The producers process the fish oil using various methods and ship the bulk oil to distributors, who purchase the bulk oil and encapsulate it, usually in gelatin capsules. In some cases, retailers purchase the capsules already made and put their own label on the bottles. Some oils are produced and encapsulated under nitrogen, while some are exposed to oxygen during their manufacture.

Most fish oil supplements found in health food stores and pharmacies contain only 30 percent omega-3 fatty acids, usually with a ratio of EPA to DHA no greater than two to one. This means that it would take thirty 1000-milligram capsules per day to match what we used in our bipolar study! This number is obviously impossible for most people to tolerate due to the daunting number of capsules to swallow, the cost, and the high likelihood of a fishy repeat. These 30 percent supplement capsules are not ideal, but until recently were the only readily available form of fish oil. The remaining 70 percent of the fish oil in these low-concentration preparations is mainly omega-9 fatty acids (such as oleic acid), some omega-6 fatty acids, cholesterol, and other lipids.

To reduce the number of capsules required per day or get a higher amount of EPA and DHA in a smaller capsule size, it is well worth the search for a more highly concentrated product. There are several high-quality concentrated fish oil supplements ranging from 50 percent omega-3 content to more than 90 percent omega-3 content.

After our study showed that fish oil could elevate and stabilize mood, many other clinicians and I began using omega-3 fish oil supplements in our clinical work. In response to the feedback we received from people taking omega-3 supplements, it became clear that many wanted to take fewer and smaller capsules, and desired a high concentration supplement without a fishy aftertaste. I approached several fish oil manufacturers and distributors urging them to produce such a supplement. No one was interested. Finally, in response to the repeated requests from people across the country, Harvard psychiatrist and fellow omega-3 researcher (and my wife) Carol A. Locke, M.D., decided to create a highly concentrated (more than 90 percent), pharmaceutical quality omega-3 supplement. She formulated the product, known as OmegaBrite, to have a high EPA to DHA ratio, and to be manufactured under nitrogen. In addition to this product, there are other high quality, pharmaceutical-grade supplements available. Table A-4 within Appendix A contains a listing of several high quality omega-3 supplements, along with their characteristics. I encourage the reader to try different supplements in order to determine which products best suit you and your family's needs.

Table 14-1 describes a number of characteristics to consider when choosing an omega-3 dietary supplement.

The source of the fish is also important. Antarctica has cleaner waters than many other regions used for fish catches. Anchovies from Antarctica are very small fish, high in omega-3 fatty acid content (and in coenzyme Q10 and other nutrients) and very low on the food chain. Using anchovies as the source has numerous advantages, including the fact that anchovy stocks are plentiful and, compared to many larger fish species, are much less prone to become depleted. Being low on the food chain and having a short life span also indicates that anchovies have far less risk of contamination with heavy metals or organic carcinogens, such as PCBs.

Distillation processes vary. Molecular distillation requires a low-temperature vacuum distillation process, which literally lifts the EPA and DHA away from the fish oil residue. This concentrating process further ensures an omega-3 supplement free of any potential contaminants.

Determining the Amount of Omega-3, DHA, and EPA in Your Supplement

Evaluating the total amount of EPA and DHA is made confusing by an FDA labeling requirement. The FDA requires that the Supplement Facts Box list amounts of omega-3 EPA and DHA,

Table 14–1: Desirable Characteristics of an Omega-3 Fatty Acid Supplement (Fish Oil)

- *Highest concentration of omega-3 fatty acids.* Supplements are available with omega-3 fatty acid concentrations ranging from 30% to more than 90%. Highly concentrated oils require fewer capsules per day and are highly purified.
- *Highest concentration of EPA per capsule.* Preliminary data suggests that EPA is the active mood agent of fish oil. EPA is also the omega-3 fatty acid that has anti-inflammatory actions and promotes heart and joint health. (Infants and pregnant or nursing women require more DHA.)
- *Highest ratio of EPA to DHA.* Preliminary data indicates that EPA is active in mood and other disorders. Very little DHA is required by an older child or adult to maintain healthy tissue concentrations. (Again, infants and pregnant or nursing women require more DHA.)
- *Low omega-6 fatty acid and saturated fat concentration.* In unconcentrated formulations, composition of the remaining non-omega-3 fatty acid in the oil becomes more important. A good brand ought to specify if any other oils are present.
- *Pharmaceutical Grade Purity.* Indicates the highest grade of purity and manufacturing quality.
- *Color and smell of oil.* Oil should be clear and light yellow in color. High-quality fish oil has a slight marine odor and either no repeat or a very mild repeat. Strong fishy odor indicates rancidity.
- *Molecular distillation.* Molecular distillation separates oil from toxins such as mercury and PCBs. Low-concentration oils may contain these toxins if they do not undergo molecular distillation. Highest-quality oils pass California's proposition 65. But oils are not required to be tested.
- *Winterization.* During the "winterization" process, oil is cooled to a low temperature, allowing saturated fats and other impurities to solidify and be removed.
- *Manufacture and encapsulation under nitrogen.* Nitrogen preserves potency by preventing oxidation and rancidity. Rancid oil smells and tastes terrible.
- *Peroxide value less than 5 at time of manufacture.* Low peroxide value indicates oil is not rancid. Lipid peroxides form when fatty acids are oxidized. This information should be available from the manufacturer.
- *Source of fish oil, including type of fish and location of catch.* Cold-water, small oily fish contain the most omega-3 fatty acids. Small species such as sardines and anchovies are shorter-lived and lower on the food chain, and therefore are also less prone to accumulate environmental pollutants. Antarctic waters are among the least polluted bodies of water on earth. These factors are particularly important in brands not purified by distillation.
- *Low cholesterol concentration.* No or very little cholesterol. Presence and concentration of cholesterol should be listed on the label.
- *No cod liver oil.* Cod liver and other fish liver oils should be avoided as the source of omega-3 fatty acids, because fish liver oil contains toxic amounts of vitamin A at higher dosages.
- *Presence of tocopherols (vitamin E) in the encapsulated oil as antioxidants.* Very small amounts of vitamin E (< 5 IU) can help prevent oxidation and preserve potency and freshness of the fish oil product.

and other ingredients based on the recommended daily serving size. Recommended serving sizes can range from one brand recommending 2 capsules per day to another brand recommending 15 capsules per day. This makes it extremely difficult to compare the amount of omega-3 EPA and DHA between brands by just looking at the Supplement Facts Box. In order to compare amounts of omega-3 per capsule between two brands, it is necessary to divide the milligram amount of omega-3 (EPA or EPA + DHA) listed in the ingredient panel by the number of capsules per serving. To further confuse the situation, omega-3 supplement capsule sizes vary from 250 mg per capsule all the way to 1200 mg per capsule. Unfortunately, the FDA does not provide a listing for the capsule size in the Supplement Facts Box on the package. Generally, one can look to the listing for total fat content to indicate approximate capsule size, since omega-3 supplements are virtually all lipids.

When comparing omega-3 content per capsule across brands, or in calculating the amount you want to use daily, take special care to determine the precise quantity of omega-3 EPA and DHA per capsule. Common additives are vitamin E or other antioxidants. If the information regarding manufacturing methods, source of the oil, or any of the other criteria are not on the box, you can call the manufacturer to acquire more information.

Flaxseed Oil

Flaxseeds, purslane, walnut, perilla, and many other somewhat exotic land-based plants contain high concentrations of the shorter-chain omega-3 fatty acid alpha-linolenic acid. Some alpha-linolenic acid can be converted in our bodies to the longer-chain omega-3s EPA and DHA. Although the scientific literature is mixed on this issue, humans may be unable to convert enough ALA to EPA and DHA to achieve optimal levels of these long-chain omega-3s.

This means that a strict vegetarian (a vegan) who eats no animal products at all will have to rely on those terrestrial sources of a possibly inferior omega-3 fatty acid. When you combine this with other potential vitamin deficiencies that often plague strict vegetarians (for example, vitamin B_{12} deficiency), and the fact that humans evolved as omnivores (eating both plants and animals), it is easy to see that many strict vegetarians are placing themselves at some risk.

Nonetheless, eating foods high in ALA is better than not receiving any omega-3 fatty acids at all. The advantages of using flaxseed oil as an omega-3 supplement include its relatively low price (in the liquid form) and its high natural concentration of alpha-linolenic acid (about 40 to 50 percent, which provides approximately 7 grams of alpha-linolenic acid per 1 tablespoon, or 15 cc, of flaxseed oil). Flaxseed oil capsules containing approximately 50 percent alpha-linolenic acid are also available, but are about the same price as fish oil capsules.

The taste of flaxseed oil, which is obtained from the plant *Linum usitatissimum*, varies from brand to brand. Very few people enjoy the taste of plain flaxseed oil, but many tolerate it. Patients in my practice have chased the liquid flaxseed oil with orange juice or chocolate milk to get rid of the taste, with fairly good results. If drinking the liquid is too repugnant, there are a number of simple recipes available that incorporate flaxseed oil (see Chapter 15).

The big drawback to flaxseed oil and other omega-3 fatty-acid–containing terrestrial plants is that ALA has not been tested in psychiatric illnesses, and there is very little data in other medical disorders. Our anecdotal experience with flaxseed oil has been mixed, and we have observed several cases of induced mania and hypomania during flaxseed oil treatment. Mania in this case refers to a condition in which a substance, such as an antidepressant, will produce an abnormal mood elevation characterized by euphoria or irritability, decreased sleep, increased energy, impulsive and dangerous behaviors, and, in severe cases, hallucinations and delusions. This finding has been observed by several of my colleagues and was previously noted by psychiatrist Donald Rudin, who published his use of flaxseed oil to treat a variety of patients in open-label studies in the 1970s and 1980s.

The liquid preparations of flaxseed oil spoil rapidly when not refrigerated, and patients who travel frequently have had logistical difficulties with the liquid flaxseed oil. Flaxseed oil capsules are a practical but more expensive alternative to the liquid.

The final word on flaxseed oil is not yet in, though studies have begun to look at it for depression. For now, concentrated fish oil is probably a better choice because of the available supportive data and greater demonstrated safety.

Indications for Using Flaxseed Oil Rather Than Fish Oil

- Inability to afford fish oil capsules; use liquid flaxseed oil (flaxseed oil capsules are about the same price as fish oil capsules)
- Strict vegetarian (vegan)
- Allergy to fish. Individuals with only shellfish allergy can often still use fish oil, but should check with their health-care provider first.
- Inability to tolerate fish oil "repeat"

Using the Omega-3 Fatty Acids for Mood Enhancement

Fish Oil

Since EPA appears to be the active mood component of fish oil, calculate the amount needed based on the concentration of EPA listed on the label. Read labels carefully, because the amount of omega-3 per serving, rather than per capsule, is listed. The recommendations listed below are estimates, since the minimum effective amount of omega-3 fatty acids remains unknown. In addition, the proper dosage appears to be highly individualized. This means that trying different amounts to find the most effective amount is crucial before giving up on the omega-3s.

Starting amount: 1.5 to 4 grams of EPA (or EPA plus DHA, if desired) per day. Use 1 gm for cardiac health, and a lower dosage range for general or mental health enhancement or for mild mood symptoms. For moderate or severe symptoms, higher amounts may be more effective.

Maintenance: Fish oil is often used long term for mood enhancement and stabilization and as part of an overall health-enhancing program. Some people elect to reduce the number of capsules once they have responded, although the so-called maintenance amount of fish oil appears to be similar to that which was initially effective. If, after lowering the amount, mood symptoms return, then return to the previously effective amount. Switching from a high-EPA brand of fish oil to a high-DHA brand has resulted in worsening depressive symptoms in some patients. If this occurs, consider returning to a high-EPA brand.

High amounts: Some people appear to require an intake of omega-3s similar to or even higher than the nearly 10 grams per day (6.2 grams EPA) that we used in our bipolar study. The highest number of grams that I have used in my practice was 12 grams of omega-3 (approximately 8 grams of EPA and 4 grams of DHA). Although this may sound like a large amount, it is still considerably less than the 14 to 19 grams of omega-3 per day that the Inuit eating a traditional diet of fish and marine mammals would receive.

Always take vitamins C and E when you are taking fish or flaxseed oil. These antioxidant vitamins preserve the omega-3s by protecting them from oxidation.

Flaxseed Oil

Whether the liquid or capsule form is used, calculate the amount of omega-3 based on the concentration of omega-3 fatty acid (alpha-linolenic acid) listed on the label.

Starting amount: 3 to 5 grams per day of alpha-linolenic acid is a reasonable starting point.

Maintenance: As with fish oil, flaxseed oil is often used long term. Usually an amount close to that which worked initially is required, but a trial of a lower amount may be a reasonable option once a response has been achieved.

High amounts: Extremely high amounts of flaxseed oil (20 to 40 grams per day and higher) have been associated with hypomania and mania. The risk of developing a hypomanic or manic episode at less than 20 grams per day is probably low. Nevertheless, close monitoring of patients receiving flaxseed oil is required, particularly if they have bipolar disorder.

If you are using flaxseeds or flaxmeal, it is important not to consume more than 2 to 3 tablespoons per day because the seed husks contain naturally occurring cyanogenic nitrates and linamarin, which can be toxic in higher doses. The cyanogenic nitrates interfere with the thyroid gland's ability to take up iodine and may lead to goiter or other thyroid problems. Immature seeds contain higher amounts of cyanogenic nitrates and glucosides and are more dangerous. Flaxseeds also contain lignans, which have mild estrogenic, antiestrogenic, and steroidlike activity. These problems are not present with flaxseed oil.

As already noted, always take vitamins C and E when you are taking fish or flaxseed oil. These antioxidant vitamins protect the omega-3s from excessive oxidation.

Potential Side Effects and Toxicity of Omega-3 Fatty Acids

Because the omega-3 fatty acids are a normal part of a diet for optimal health, it is not surprising that there are very few side effects associated with even enormous dosages of supplements. Probably the best way to think about this issue is to split the side effects into potentially medically serious side effects, versus those that are more of a nuisance, without serious medical consequences.

Gastrointestinal Side Effects

Among the nuisance side effects, gastrointestinal symptoms, which include rare nausea and occasional diarrhea, are the most common. The severity of these side effects is generally proportional to the dosage. It is not surprising that a high dosage of any oil (including fish or flaxseed oil) can cause gastrointestinal side effects. Fortunately, there are some useful remedies that eliminate or reduce these problems.

Regarding any of the gastrointestinal side effects, taking less oil at one time will reduce or eliminate the side effects. Take the omega-3 with meals. Everyone is different in respect to how much omega-3 fatty acid can be taken without gastrointestinal side effects. Some people can take a large amount of fish or flaxseed oil all at once and have no side effects. Others are sensitive to even small amounts. Most people do well taking the oils twice per day, with breakfast and dinner. Others prefer to take the bulk of the oil at night, before going to bed. And still others take the oil three or four times per day to reduce any gastrointestinal side effects. Obviously the higher the concentration of omega-3 in a supplement, the fewer capsules and the less oil you will have to consume.

There is no evidence that the effectiveness of omega-3 oils varies if you take the oil once, twice, or more times per day. Splitting the dosage up is mainly for convenience or to reduce gastrointestinal side effects.

Another strategy for reducing nausea associated with omega-3 oils is to use a supplement without a fishy taste or odor. Some of the higher-concentration oils have little or no fishy taste associated with them. Some people simply take their omega-3 supplement with food to avoid nausea. Others have had success with gingerroot capsules to reduce nausea. Although there is no clinical study demonstrating that gingerroot will reduce nausea from omega-3s, gingerroot has been used for centuries in traditional Chinese medicine to treat gastrointestinal symptoms.

Strategies to reduce the fishy aftertaste with omega-3 supplements are similar to those used to reduce nausea, particularly that of taking smaller amounts of oil in each dose and using the highest-concentration, least-fishy-tasting supplement. I have patients who take their omega-3 supplement with orange juice or chocolate milk, strong-tasting beverages that seem to reduce the fishy aftertaste of some omega-3 supplements. Taking most of the oil at night will also reduce the fishy aftertaste problem, since almost all of the oil will be passed from the stomach during sleep.

Many of these strategies also reduce or eliminate the diarrhea occasionally associated with large amounts of omega-3 supplements. Taking food or other dietary supplements, which may improve fat absorption, could also reduce diarrhea. A patient of mine has successfully used daikon radish, an Asian vegetable, reported to improve digestion after a fatty meal.

Hypervitaminosis A: Warning

Hypervitaminosis A occurs when the level of the fat-soluble vitamin A is excessively high in the blood, leading to hair loss, arthritis-like symptoms, liver problems, and other serious symptoms; Hypervitaminosis A may be the result of using too many vitamin A supplements, or taking excessive amounts of cod liver oil which contains high levels of vitamin A. To achieve some of the higher quantities of omega-3 fatty acids described in this book, it could be potentially dangerous to use cod liver oil, since vitamin A could rise to a dangerous level. Most fish oil sold as dietary supplements comes from the muscles of the fish, which have much lower vitamin A levels than the liver. I advise not using cod liver oil or the oil from any other fish liver as a source of omega-3 fatty acids.

Impaired Platelet Function

Platelets are in the bloodstream to help with blood clotting if an injury occurs. At the site of tissue injury, chemicals of the inflammatory process are released, which cause the platelets to clump together and start the process of wound healing. If the platelets are overactive, they can clump together inside the wall of a blood vessel and promote atherosclerosis or even cause a sudden blockage of a blood vessel, which can lead to stroke or heart attack. Aspirin helps prevent heart attacks by inhibiting platelets from sticking together. This is usually beneficial, unless the platelets are inhibited too strongly. If the platelets will not stick together, abnormal bleeding can occur. (This is sometimes a serious problem with aspirin therapy.) Like aspirin, omega-3 fatty acids also inhibit platelets from sticking together, but in a slightly different way that does not affect normal blood clotting and wound healing. The partial blockade of platelet aggregation by omega-3 fatty acids is only one of the ways these oils help reduce the risk of heart disease. Fortunately, the omega-3 fatty acids do not block platelet action to the extent that aspirin does, and bleeding has not been reported with fish oil. However, if you are receiving high-dose aspirin or ibuprofen, or another drug in this class, or if you are taking other blood thinners, such as warfarin (Coumadin), you should check with your health-care provider before starting an omega-3 fatty acid supplement. Most likely, no dangerous interaction will occur, particularly at low dosages of omega-3s.

Drug Interactions

The antiplatelet action of high-dose omega-3 oils could theoretically intensify the anticoagulant effects of warfarin, high-dose aspirin, and other blood thinners. However, there has never been a case reported of abnormal or excessive bleeding resulting from omega-3 supplements, so the chances of a drug interaction are probably quite low. Nonetheless, consult with your physician if you are taking any of these medications.

One other potential drug interaction is with the anti-obesity drug orlistat (Xenical). Orlistat reduces the absorption of all fats and potentially could diminish the absorption of omega-3 fatty acids. If the orlistat and the omega-3 supplements are taken many hours apart, this may be less of a problem.

Antioxidants and Vitamin Supplements

It is essential to have abundant amounts of antioxidants in your body when taking omega-3 supplements or increasing the omega-3s in your diet. The best way to get these antioxidants is in food and by taking selected supplemental vitamins and minerals. A supplement may not have the same positive effect as whole food. This is probably because plants contain other useful phytochemicals beyond the known antioxidants that we have identified. Many of these phytochemicals appear to work synergistically with each other, but have not been well studied.

By using foods to obtain needed substances, we are absorbing many different and powerful types of antioxidants, such as lycopene and rosmarnic acid. Vitamin E in the form of gamma-tocopherol is found in soybeans and nuts. Foods that are deeply pigmented contain flavonoids, which are water-soluble and often highly colored antioxidants. Examples are lutein in dark-green kale; lycopene in tomatoes; beta-carotene in sweet potatoes, squash, carrots, and other orange fruits; and zeaxanthin in pepper. Deeply pigmented fruits such as blueberries, cantaloupe, and kiwi contain other antioxidants. Grapes and grape leaves contain reservatol, and grape seeds contain the antioxidant proanthocyanidin. Coenzyme Q10, a potent antioxidant in every cell, is found in spinach, peanuts, and sardines. Green tea and even black tea contain important antioxidants called tannins, which are polymers of phenolic compounds.

Antioxidants capture free radicals (highly reactive compounds with "free" electrons), which are dangerous to the omega-3 essential fatty acids. The more double bonds the omega-3 has, the more vulnerable it is to oxidation. Oxidation of omega-3 fatty acids has two negative consequences: (1) destruction of the omega-3s and loss of their biological activity, and (2) the production of lipid peroxides, which are highly chemically reactive compounds that can damage cell membranes further.

Beyond obtaining antioxidants in food, it may be necessary to take 1000 milligrams per day of vitamin C and 800 IU (International Units) of vitamin E per day. Recent data suggest that the combination of vitamins C and E may be superior to either one alone. It has been suggested that the vitamin C regenerates any oxidized vitamin E. These vitamins have very different but complementary chemical properties. Vitamin C is water soluble and diffuses into the watery center of the cell, known as the cytoplasm, and into the extracellular fluid surrounding the cell. Vitamin E is fat soluble and remains within the lipid-rich cell membranes protecting the omega-3.

Magnesium, selenium, zinc, coenzyme Q10, the B vitamins, folic acid, pyridoxine, and nicotinamide all work with vitamins C and E to protect omega-3 fatty acids and other fragile cellular biochemicals.

In summary I recommend on a daily basis the following:

- Vitamin E: 800 IU (International Units) per day of natural alpha-tocopherols (organic sources if affordable)
- Vitamin C: 1000 milligrams per day
- A good general multivitamin that includes magnesium, selenium, zinc, B vitamins (B_{12} and B_6, folic acid, pyridoxine, nicotinamide), and coenzyme Q10.

Helping the Omega-3s Work Better: Exercise, Relaxation, and Positive Cognitive Techniques

We live in a stressful world. Increasing the amount of omega-3s in your diet through the Omega-3 Renewal Plan can help provide the basic biological foundation of mental health, adaptation to stress, and happiness. And there are other changes you can make to enhance your mental and physical health. Along with increasing omega-3, exercise is probably the most powerful way to enhance health, longevity, and happiness. There are many excellent forms of exercise, but the major factor in determining the success of any program is perseverance. Daily exercise must become part of your life's routine.

Another way to reduce the negative effects of stress on health is to perform daily relaxation exercises, such as meditation. There are also several types of simple but rapidly effective cognitive exercises that you can perform yourself or with a therapist; they help enhance mood and self-esteem. Most of these exercises involve changing the way you think about yourself by using specific cognitive techniques performed over and over again, such as positive self-statements or visualization.

Plug Into the Omega-3 Connection

The purpose of this book is to make more people aware of the remarkable group of essential nutrients known as the omega-3 fatty acids and their vital importance to every cell in the human body. Widespread omega-3 depletion is reducing the quality and length of the lives of our children and ourselves. By restoring the diet and nutrition of our evolutionary ancestors, we may be able to reduce the prevalence of many modern diseases, such as depression and heart disease, and recreate the biochemical environment inside our bodies that is associated with optimal general and emotional health. I hope the delicious recipes and ordering information in Chapter 15 will help you achieve this goal.

15

Recipes: Good Health and Good Taste

೨ Now that you understand the valuable role omega-3 fats play in health, the logical next step is to find ways to include more of these beneficial fats in your diet. For most Americans, this is a difficult task because the list of omega-3-rich foods is fairly short: salmon (and other fatty fish), purslane, flaxseed, walnuts, flaxseed oil, omega-3-enriched eggs, wild game meats, and, to a lesser extent, canola oil. Start working some of these foods into meals, for example, by sprinkling some ground flaxseed on cereal in the morning, cooking with canola oil instead of corn or safflower oil, or adding an omega-3-enriched egg to a favorite muffin recipe. Then build from there, gradually shifting the balance of omega-3 and omega-6 polyunsaturated fats to healthier levels.

Although most people eat a diet far richer in omega-6 than omega-3 fats, perhaps even ten to twenty times richer, a 1 to 1 ratio is probably ideal. It is important to remember that excessive consumption of some wild fish can result in potential toxicity from mercury and certain organic chemical contaminants from industrial pollution. For this reason, and because of the general lack of readily available omega-3-rich foods, most Americans require omega-3 supplements to augment their diet if they want to achieve mood-elevating levels of omega-3 fatty acids in their bodies.

To help in the effort toward a healthier diet, we've developed twenty simple and delicious omega-3-boosting recipes—everything from appetizers to salads to entrees. Enjoy some omega-3s at breakfast with delicious pancakes made with ground flaxseed. They are rich in omega-3s and contain a generous amount of fiber and iron. For supper, try the honey-walnut roasted salmon, a simple-to-fix baked fish that has both the animal-based long-chain omega-3s (EPA, DHA) and the plant-based shorter chain omega-3, alpha-linolenic acid (ALA). Each recipe has been analyzed for several nutrients, with an emphasis on the amount and type of fat per serving. The complete fat breakdown includes a listing of the total grams of fat—saturated fat, monounsaturated fat, and polyunsaturated fat, and then a further breakdown of polyunsaturated fat that includes the omega-3 fats (EPA, DHA, ALA) as well as the amount of omega-6 fat.

Although the ratio of omega-6 to omega-3 fats is important, do not agonize over all of these fat numbers. They simply provide a nutritional snapshot of how each recipe can contribute to your omega-3-rich eating plan and help you shift the balance of omega-3s in your diet to higher levels. Of course, omega-3 fats are only one part of a healthy diet, so we've included information about other major nutrition concerns, such as calories, fiber, cholesterol, iron, and sodium. Keep in mind that these recipes are just a starting point, albeit a delicious one, that lets you see how easily flaxseed, walnuts, salmon, and all the other foods rich in omega-3s can be worked into meals. There's really no limit on the amount of these key fats you can include in your diet. Start by stocking the pantry with omega-3-rich foods (a list of where you can buy these products follows the recipes), and before you know it, you'll be well on your way to an omega-3-rich style of eating.

People have asked me whether or not the fragile omega-3 fatty acids are destroyed during the preparation and cooking of omega-3-rich foods. Certainly, using an oil for frying would likely destroy most, if not all, of the omega-3s. However, when the omega-3 is within the food, whether it is a salmon steak or a flax muffin, it is at least partially protected by the lower temperature inside the food relative to the oven or pan. Some omega-3 is likely lost, but most is probably preserved. Eating sushi or sashimi, or Japanese raw fish, would obviously circumvent this issue.

EVERYDAY DISHES

Salads

Mixed Greens with Toasted Walnut Vinaigrette

8 SERVINGS

Because flaxseed oil is delicate and doesn't do so well in cooking, vinaigrettes and salad dressing are a perfect way to include more of this healthy oil in your diet. Here we've added toasted walnuts to the mix to increase the alpha-linolenic acid content of the dressing even further and to complement the nutty overtones of flax oil. A small amount of canola oil is used to help temper the intense flavor of flaxseed oil.

> 2 garlic cloves, peeled and halved
> eight ½-inch-thick slices French bread baguette
> ½ cup sherry or red wine vinegar
> ½ teaspoon freshly ground pepper
> ½ teaspoon salt
> 2 tablespoons minced shallot or red onion
> 6 tablespoons flaxseed or walnut oil
> 2 tablespoons canola oil
> 2 tablespoons finely chopped walnuts, toasted
> 6 cups salad greens
> 1 cup watercress
> 1 cup chopped purslane

Preheat the oven to 375 degrees.

Rub the garlic on one side of each slice of bread, and place the bread on a baking sheet. Bake for 4 to 5 minutes on each side, or until crisp and golden.

Combine the sherry and the next six ingredients in a bowl. Whisk well. Combine the greens, watercress, and purslane in a large salad bowl. Drizzle the vinaigrette over the greens and toss.

Serve each salad with one slice of garlic toast.

Cooking tip. Walnuts and blue cheese are a great flavor pair, so a small amount of crumbled blue cheese—about ½ ounce per salad—will give a nice richness to this salad and will add just under 3 grams of saturated fat.

Nutrition profile. 1 cup of greens, 1 garlic toast, and 2 tablespoons of vinaigrette:

Calories, 171; fat, 15.4 g; (1.8 g saturated, 4.6 g monounsaturated, 8.3 g polyunsaturated); protein, 1.7 g; carbohydrate, 7.8 g; fiber, 1 g; cholesterol, 0 mg; sodium, 200 mg.
Omega-3s: ALA, 1.8 g; EPA, none; DHA, none.
Omega-6: 6.5 g.
Ratio of omega-6 to omega-3: 3.6.

Tabbouleh with Walnuts

SIX 1-CUP SERVINGS

This Middle Eastern salad is usually made with lots of parsley and olive oil. Here we've substituted some purslane for part of the parsley, changed the oil, and added some toasted walnuts for a triple punch of the plant-based omega-3 fat, alpha-linolenic acid. If you can't find purslane, substitute parsley. Look for bulgur—wheat kernels that are steamed, dried, and then cracked—in the rice/grain aisle of the supermarket or in a health-food store.

1 cup fine or medium bulgur
1 cup boiling water
1½ cups finely chopped fresh purslane
1½ cups finely chopped fresh parsley
2 cups chopped, seeded tomato
1 cup thinly sliced green onion (including green tops)
½ cup finely chopped fresh mint
¼ cup finely chopped walnuts
2 tablespoons flaxseed or walnut oil
1 tablespoon canola oil
¼ cup fresh lemon juice
1 teaspoon salt

Combine the bulgur and boiling water in a large bowl and stir well. Let stand 30 minutes, or until the water is absorbed. Add the purslane and the next 5 ingredients to the cooked bulgur.

Combine the oils and the remaining ingredients, and pour over the tabbouleh.

Serve at room temperature or chilled.

Cooking tip. Both walnut and flaxseed oil are strong flavored, so a small amount of the more neutral canola oil helps to temper their intensity. But you can omit the canola oil if you like and use all walnut or flaxseed oil.

Nutrition profile. 1 cup:

Calories, 196; fat, 10.5 g (1 g saturated, 3.2 g monounsaturated, 5.7 g polyunsaturated); protein, 4.9 g; carbohydrate, 24 g; fiber, 6.1 g; cholesterol, 0 mg; sodium, 219 mg.
Omega-3s: ALA, 3.2 g; EPA, none; DHA, none.
Omega-6: 2.7 g.
Ratio of omega-6 to omega-3: 0.8.

Pasta Primavera Salad with Pesto

Six 1½-cup servings

Purslane, a richer source of alpha-linolenic acid than any other commercially available leafy green, is a perfect herb for pesto. But the stems can be sour, so just use the leaves. If you can't find purslane, replace it with parsley. You'll still have a good dose of alpha-linolenic acid from the walnuts and flaxseed oil.

2 cups fresh cilantro leaves
1 cup fresh purslane leaves
¼ cup fresh parsley sprigs
½ cup walnuts
¼ cup freshly grated Parmesan cheese
1 teaspoon salt
4 garlic cloves
¼ cup flaxseed or walnut oil

2 cups chopped, seeded tomato
⅔ cup shredded carrot
1 yellow pepper, sliced into small strips
8 cups cooked penne or other cooked pasta (shells, macaroni, bow ties)

Place the first seven ingredients in a food processor, and process until smooth. With the processor on, slowly pour the oil through the food chute, and process until well blended. Toss with the rest of the ingredients.

Cooking tip. Make lots of this pesto in the summer months while purslane is in season, and freeze the leftovers. Try the pesto as a topping for grilled chicken or fish or as a sandwich spread, or just spread it on some toasted French bread as an appetizer. Buy preshredded carrots and shredded Parmesan to save time.

Nutrition profile. 1½ cups:

Calories, 453; fat, 18.8 g (2.2 g saturated, 4.0 g monounsaturated, 10.2 g polyunsaturated); protein, 13.9 g; carbohydrate, 58.1 g; fiber, 4.6 g; cholesterol, 6 mg; sodium, 520 mg.
Omega-3s: ALA, 6.1 g; EPA, none; DHA, none.
Omega-6: 2.8 g.
Ratio of omega-6 to omega-3: 0.5.

Entrees

Honey-Walnut Roasted Salmon

4 SERVINGS

This recipe produces a double punch of omega-3s since salmon is one of the richest sources of beneficial EPA and DHA and two of the ingredients in the topping—walnuts and purslane—are rich in alpha-linolenic acid, the plant-based shorter chain omega-3. Wild salmon usually has larger amounts of omega-3s than farm-raised salmon in the United States; but farm-raised salmon has less chance of being contaminated with environmental toxins.

1 slice firm white bread
3 tablespoons chopped fresh purslane or parsley
2 cloves garlic, minced
⅓ cup finely chopped walnuts
1 teaspoon minced fresh lemon zest
four 6-ounce salmon fillets, about 1¼ inches thick at
   the thickest part
2 tablespoons honey
½ teaspoon coarse or regular salt
¼ teaspoon fresh ground black pepper
1 teaspoon canola oil

Preheat the oven to 425 degrees.

Break the bread into pieces. Place the bread in a food processor or blender and process to form fresh bread crumbs. Combine the bread crumbs, purslane, garlic, walnuts and zest in a flat, shallow bowl. Brush the top and sides of each fillet with ½ tablespoon honey. Sprinkle each with salt and black pepper, and dip it into the bread crumb mixture, pressing down firmly to make the bread crumbs stick to the top and sides. Place the fish skin side down in an 11- by 7-inch baking dish brushed with canola oil or on a lightly oiled baking sheet.

Bake for 15 minutes, or until the fish flakes easily when tested with a fork.

Cooking tip. Salmon fillets vary in thickness. Measure the fillet at its thickest point, and estimate about 10 minutes of roasting time for each 1 inch of thickness.

Nutrition profile. 1 fillet:

Calories, 368; fat, 18.4 g (2.6 g saturated, 5.7 g monounsaturated, 8.6 g polyunsaturated); protein, 35.9 g; carbohydrate, 14.6 g; fiber, 0.5 g; cholesterol, 94 mg; iron, 1.8 mg; sodium, 402 mg.
Omega-3s: ALA, 1.0 g; EPA, 1.0 g; DHA, 2.0 g.
Omega-6: 1.2 g.
Ratio of omega-6 to omega-3: 0.6.

Cracked Pepper Salmon

4 SERVINGS

Salmon is one of the richest sources of beneficial EPA and DHA.

2 tablespoons cracked or coarsely ground black pepper
1 tablespoon Italian seasoning
½ teaspoon salt
¼ teaspoon garlic powder
four 6-ounce salmon fillets, about ¾ inch thick at the thickest
  point
2 tablespoons all-purpose flour
1 tablespoon canola oil

Combine the first four ingredients in a small bowl. Rub the salmon with the mixture and dredge the salmon in the flour.
Pour the canola oil into a large skillet over medium-high heat. Add the salmon, and sauté for 4 minutes on each side, or until the fish flakes easily when tested with a fork.

Cooking tip. It's best to use thinner fillets for the skillet because they cook more evenly.

Nutrition profile. 1 fillet:

Calories, 300; fat, 14.5 g (2 g saturated, 5.6 g monounsaturated, 5.4 g polyunsaturated); protein, 34.7 g; carbohydrate, 6.3 g; fiber, 1.3 g; cholesterol, 94 mg; sodium, 370 mg.
Omega-3s: ALA, 1.0 g; EPA, 1.0 g; DHA, 2 g.
Omega-6: 2.0 g.
Ratio of omega-6 to omega-3: 0.5.

New Orleans Trout Sandwich

6 SERVINGS

This version of the popular New Orleans sandwich uses trout, which carries a generous supply of EPA and DHA, instead of catfish. (All va-

rieties of trout contain omega-3 fats, but if you can find lake trout, it is a bit richer in these fats than the brook or rainbow trout varieties.)

⅓ cup yellow corn meal
3 tablespoons all-purpose flour
1 tablespoon Cajun seasoning
six 6-ounce trout fillets, skinned
1 tablespoon canola oil
6 long 2-ounce sandwich rolls
leaf lettuce
sliced red tomatoes

Combine the corn meal, flour, and Cajun seasoning in a shallow dish. Dredge the trout in the mixture.

Place 1½ teaspoons of oil in a large nonstick skillet over medium-high heat. Add 3 trout fillets, and cook for 2 to 3 minutes on each side, or until the fish flakes easily when tested with a fork. Remove the fish from the pan and keep warm. Repeat the procedure with the remaining 1½ teaspoons of oil and trout.

Place each piece of fish on a sandwich roll with lettuce, tomato, and any condiment of choice.

Cooking tip. Since canola oil mayonnaise carries 1 gram of ALA per tablespoon, you might consider making a spicy Cajun-style sauce for this sandwich. Mix together and chill the following ingredients: 6 tablespoons canola oil mayonnaise, 2 tablespoons coarse ground mustard, 2 tablespoons sweet pickle relish, 2 tablespoons chopped red onion, 1 teaspoon hot sauce, and ¼ teaspoon black pepper.

Nutrition profile. 1 sandwich:

Calories, 463; fat, 15.2 g (2.2 g saturated, 5.5 g monounsaturated, 4.8 g polyunsaturated); protein, 42.4 g; carbohydrate, 41.4 g; fiber, 1.7 g; cholesterol, 107 mg; sodium, 686 mg.
Omega-3s: ALA, 1.1 g; EPA, 0.85 g; DHA, 1.86 g.
Omega-6: 2.9 g.
Ratio of omega-6 to omega-3: 0.76.

Grilled Teriyaki Tuna

4 SERVINGS

Teriyaki is a Japanese term describing food marinated in a mixture of soy sauce, sake (rice wine) or sherry, sugar, ginger, and spices. Here we've used tuna, but you could easily substitute another omega-3-rich fish such as salmon.

⅓ cup soy sauce
3 tablespoons brown sugar
3 tablespoons sherry or sake
1 tablespoon peeled, minced gingerroot
¼ teaspoon red pepper flakes
1 clove garlic, minced
four 6-ounce tuna steaks, about ¾ inch thick each
8 green onions (optional)
1 teaspoon canola oil

Combine the first six ingredients in a large zip-top bag. Add the tuna and green onions if you are using them. Zip the bag shut, and marinate in the refrigerator for 30 minutes, turning the bag periodically.

Remove the tuna and onions from the marinade, and pat them dry. Reserve the marinade.

Brush a grill or an indoor grill pan with canola oil. Place the tuna on the grill over medium-hot coals or on the pan over medium to medium-high heat. Cook 4 minutes on each side until the tuna is medium rare, or to the desired degree of doneness, basting occasionally with the reserved marinade. Place the onions on the grill and cook for 2 to 4 minutes, or until they are softened and partially charred.

Cooking tip. To broil the tuna steaks, preheat the oven, and place the steaks on a broiler pan brushed with canola oil; cooking times are the same. For thicker (1-inch) tuna steaks, cook for 5 to 6 minutes per side.

Nutrition profile. 1 tuna steak and 2 green onions:

Calories, 314; fat, 9.6 g (2.2 g saturated, 3 g monounsaturated, 3.2 g polyunsaturated); protein, 41.2 g; carbohydrate, 11 g; fiber, 0.7 g; cholesterol, 65 mg; sodium, 1179 mg.
Omega-3s: ALA, 0.1 g; EPA, 0.7 g; DHA, 2.0 g.
Omega-6: 0.7 g.
Ratio of omega-6 to omega-3: 0.3.

Tuna Burgers

4 SERVINGS

The omega-3 content of different canned tuna varies considerably; albacore tuna is the richest source of the beneficial fats. Because of the risk of exposure to environmental pollution, adults probably should not eat more than one can of tuna per week.

> 2 slices rye bread (about 2 ounces)
> one 12-ounce can albacore tuna packed in water, drained
> ¼ cup sliced green onion
> 2 tablespoons finely diced celery
> ⅓ cup chopped fresh parsley
> 1 tablespoon fresh lemon juice
> ¼ teaspoon cayenne
> ¼ teaspoon salt
> 2 omega-3-rich eggs, lightly beaten
> 1 tablespoon canola oil
> 4 sourdough sandwich rolls

Break the bread into pieces and place in a food processor or blender. Pulse several times to form bread crumbs. Combine the bread crumbs, tuna, green onion, and celery in a bowl. In another bowl, combine the next five ingredients. Stir them into the tuna mixture, and form the mixture into four equal-sized patties.

Heat the oil in a large nonstick skillet over medium to medium-high heat. Add the patties, and cook 4 minutes. Carefully turn the patties over, and cook 4 minutes more, or until golden. Serve on the sandwich rolls with a condiment of choice and extras such as lettuce and tomato, if desired.

Cooking tip. These fish cakes can be made with canned salmon. Use a tomato-based seafood cocktail sauce for a condiment. If you can afford a little extra fat, combine and chill 3 tablespoons of canola oil mayonnaise, 3 tablespoons of plain yogurt, 1 tablespoon of chopped fresh dill, and 1 crushed garlic clove to make a dill-garlic mayonnaise to serve with this burger.

Nutrition profile. 1 tuna burger:

Calories, 328; fat, 8.8 g (1.4 g saturated, 3.8 g monounsaturated, 2.4 g polyunsaturated); protein, 31 g; carbohydrate, 31.7 g; fiber, 2.4 g; cholesterol, 131 mg; sodium, 823 mg.
Omega-3s: ALA, 1.3 g; EPA, 0.26 g; DHA, 0.92 g.
Omega-6: 1.31 g.
Ratio of omega-6 to omega-3: 0.82.

Cowboy Quesadillas

4 SERVINGS

Buffalo meat is low in fat, low in saturated fat, low in cholesterol, and has higher levels of alpha-linolenic acid than domestic red meat. Some supermarkets, particularly in larger cities, sell ground buffalo meat. It's also becoming easy to order by mail. Check out our products page.

1 tablespoon canola oil
¾ pound ground buffalo meat
½ cup chopped yellow onion
½ teaspoon chili powder
½ teaspoon salt
½ cup bottled roasted red peppers, chopped
½ cup chopped yellow or red tomato
1 cup cooked pinto beans, partially mashed
1 teaspoon diced chipotle pepper canned in adobo sauce
1 tablespoon fresh lime juice
2 tablespoons minced fresh cilantro or parsley
eight 8-inch flour tortillas

¼ cup fancy shredded part-skim mozarella or reduced-fat
   cheddar cheese
canola oil
fresh or bottled salsa

Heat 2 teaspoons of the canola oil in a nonstick skillet over
medium heat. Add the ground buffalo, and sauté until it is fully
cooked, about 6 to 10 minutes. Remove the meat from the pan,
and add the remaining canola oil. Add the onion, and sauté 1 to 2
minutes, until the onion begins to soften. Stir in the chili powder
and salt; cook 30 seconds. Add the cooked buffalo, the red pepper, and the next five ingredients. Cook gently for 3 to 4 minutes.
Remove from the heat and keep the mixture warm.

Place a nonstick skillet brushed with canola oil over medium
heat. Add one tortilla to the pan, and top it with 2 tablespoons of
cheese. Spoon ½ cup of the buffalo mixture over the cheese; top
with another tortilla. Cook for 3 minutes, pressing down with a
spatula until the cheese melts. Turn carefully and cook until
thoroughly heated (about 1 minute).

Repeat the procedure with the remaining tortillas, cheese, and
buffalo mixture.

Cut each quesadilla into quarters, and serve with salsa.

Cooking tip. When you're trying to eat less cheese (less saturated fat) the "fancy"-style shred with its smaller pieces helps to
cover a larger surface area with a smaller amount. Chipotle peppers (smoked jalapeños) canned in adobo sauce can be found
with the Mexican foods in your supermarket. Substitute 1 teaspoon of fresh minced jalapeño for the chipotle, if desired. Omit
the hot peppers if you don't like spicy food.

Nutrition profile. 1 quesadilla plus 2 tablespoons of salsa:

Calories, 430; fat, 9.2 g (3.7 g saturated, 2.9 g monounsaturated, 1.7 g
polyunsaturated); protein, 22.5 g; carbohydrate, 66.9 g; fiber, 6.1 g;
cholesterol, 81 mg; iron, 2.1 mg; sodium, 1,125 mg; calcium, 231 mg.
Omega-3s: ALA, 0.7 g; EPA, none; DHA, none.
Omega-6: 1.0 g.
Ratio of omega-6 to omega-3: 1.4.

Bistro Roasted Venison Tenderloin

8 SERVINGS

Wild game meats such as venison are low in fat and contain higher levels of alpha-linolenic acid than domestic red meats. Researchers suspect that a wild and varied diet and a "free-to-roam" lifestyle contribute to this healthier nutrition profile.

¼ cup stone-ground mustard
2 tablespoons brown sugar
1 tablespoon red wine vinegar
2 garlic gloves, crushed
½ teaspoon coarsely ground pepper
one 2-pound venison tenderloin
1 teaspoon canola oil
2 tablespoons brown sugar
1 tablespoon red wine vinegar
½ cup fat-free beef broth
¼ cup dry red wine
¼ cup water
¼ cup minced shallot or red onion
1 tablespoon chopped fresh thyme

Combine the first five ingredients in a large zip-top plastic bag. Add the venison, and seal the bag. Marinate in the refrigerator overnight, turning the bag periodically. Remove the venison from the bag and pat it dry. Reserve leftover marinade.

Preheat the oven to 375 degrees.

Place the venison, brushed lightly with canola oil, in a small baking dish. Insert a meat thermometer into the thickest portion of the venison. Bake for 35 to 40 minutes, or until the thermometer registers 160 degrees (slightly pink) or until desired degree of doneness. Let the venison stand 10 minutes before slicing, and save any drippings from the pan.

Just before taking the venison out of the oven, combine the reserved marinade, the brown sugar and the next five ingredients in a small saucepan. Bring to a boil. Reduce the heat to medium and cook 10 to 15 minutes. Stir in the pan drippings and fresh thyme, and serve with the venison.

Cooking tip. Because it's much leaner than most other red meats, wild game meat, like venison, can be easily overcooked. Check your oven temperature carefully and keep to the specified cooking time.

Nutrition profile. 1 serving (about 3 ounces of venison plus 2 tablespoons of sauce):

Calories, 181; fat, 3.7 g (1.1 g saturated, 1.4 g monounsaturated, 0.7 g polyunsaturated); protein, 26.7 g; carbohydrate, 6.5 g; fiber, 0.2 g; cholesterol, 96 mg; sodium, 160 mg.
Omega-3s: ALA, 0.1 g; EPA, none; DHA, none.
Omega-6: 0.5 g.
Ratio of omega-6 to omega-3: 5.0.

Mediterranean Frittata

6 SERVINGS

The bulk of the beneficial fat in this easy-to-prepare meatless main dish comes from eggs, so be sure to buy a brand that is rich in omega-3s. Feta cheese, which contributes a tiny amount of saturated fat, is optional but adds a lot of flavor.

1 tablespoon canola oil
1 cup coarsely chopped red onion
2 cups thinly sliced Yukon gold or red potato
1 teaspoon salt, divided
¼ teaspoon black pepper
6 omega-3-rich eggs
½ cup chopped fresh purslane or spinach
½ cup sliced green onion
1 teaspoon chopped fresh or ½ teaspoon dried oregano
1 teaspoon chopped fresh or ½ teaspoon dried basil
6 Kalamata olives, pitted and chopped
1 ounce feta or goat cheese, crumbled (optional)

Heat the oil in a 10-inch cast-iron or nonstick skillet over medium heat. Add the red onion, and sauté 5 minutes. Layer the potato slices over the onion, and sprinkle with ½ teaspoon salt and black pepper. Cover the pan, reduce the heat to medium low, and cook 10 minutes, or until the potatoes are tender.

Combine the remaining ½ teaspoon salt, the eggs, purslane, green onion, and herbs; stir well with a whisk. Pour the egg mixture over the potatoes, and sprinkle with the olives and cheese. Cook over medium-low heat 15 to 20 minutes, or until almost set. Place the pan under the broiler for 2 to 3 minutes, until the top is browned and the eggs are completely cooked.

Nutrition profile. 1 wedge:

Calories, 169; fat, 9.1 g (2.6 g saturated, 5.9 g monounsaturated, 1.5 g polyunsaturated); protein, 8.7 g; carbohydrate, 21.2 g; fiber, 2.4 g; cholesterol, 221 mg; sodium, 551 mg.
Omega-3s: ALA, 0.4 g; EPA, 0.05 g; DHA, 0.15 g.
Omega-6: 0.5 g.
Ratio of omega-6 to omega-3: 0.8.

Desserts and Snacks

Cranberry-Apple Crisp

8 SERVINGS

Fruit crisps typically have a butter-laden topping that is crunchy. Here we've replaced the saturated fat of butter with the healthier canola oil. To help regain some of the crispness lost in that switch, we've added wheat germ and chopped walnuts. The walnuts and flaxseed meal in the topping contribute a generous portion of alpha-linolenic acid.

    4 cups peeled, thinly sliced Rome apple or other baking apple
    1 cup fresh or frozen cranberries
    3 tablespoons apple cider
    1 tablespoon brown sugar
    1 tablespoon all-purpose flour

½ cup all-purpose flour
¼ cup flaxseed meal (ground flaxseeds)
¼ cup finely chopped walnut
2 tablespoons wheat germ
⅛ teaspoon salt
¼ teaspoon cinnamon
3 tablespoons canola oil

Preheat the oven to 375 degrees.

Combine the apples, cranberries, cider, sugar, and 1 table-spoon of flour in a bowl. Mix well. Place the apple mixture in a large oval gratin dish or an 11- by 7-inch baking dish.

Combine the ½ cup of flour and the flaxseed meal. Add wal-nuts, wheat germ, salt, and cinnamon; mix well. Stir in the oil until the mixture resembles coarse crumbs. (Rub the topping gently with your hands to make uniform crumbs.) Sprinkle the topping mixture evenly over the fruit, and bake for 35 to 45 min-utes, or until it is crisp and bubbly. Serve warm.

Cooking tip. Try other combinations of fresh fruit, such as peaches and blackberries, with this same topping. To keep the topping crisp, reheat leftovers in the oven rather than in the mi-crowave.

Nutrition profile. ⅛ of a crisp:

Calories, 177; fat, 9.1 g (0.8 g saturated, 3.8 g monounsaturated, 4.0 g polyunsaturated); protein, 2.9 g; carbohydrate, 22.7 g; fiber, 3 g; cholesterol, 0 mg; sodium, 38 mg.
Omega-3s: ALA, 2.1 g; EPA, none; DHA, none.
Omega-6: 2.8 g.
Ratio of omega-6 to omega-3: 1.3.

Maple-Walnut Granola

5 CUPS

Although they're not a typical ingredient in most granolas, walnuts are the nuts richest in alpha-linolenic acid (ALA). Here we've paired them with a small amount of whole flaxseed to boost the ALA even further. Don't be tempted to replace the canola oil with flaxseed oil, however. Flaxseed oil is delicate, and the long baking time might cause it to break down.

4½ cups regular oats
1 cup coarsely chopped walnuts
1 teaspoon ground cinnamon
1 teaspoon salt
⅔ cup maple syrup
2 tablespoons honey
⅓ cup water
2 tablespoons canola oil
¼ cup flaxseeds
½ cup chopped dried fruit (such as raisins, cherries, dates)

Preheat the oven to 325 degrees.

Combine the oats, walnuts, cinnamon, and salt in a bowl, and mix well. In a small pan, combine the syrup, honey, water, and oil. Bring to a boil, remove from the heat, and stir in the flaxseeds. Pour the hot mixture over the oat mixture, stirring well to coat.

Spoon the mixture onto a baking sheet brushed lightly with canola oil, and spread evenly. Bake for 35 to 40 minutes, or until the granola is lightly toasted, stirring periodically. Remove from the oven, and stir in the dried fruit. Cool completely. Store in an airtight container to keep crisp.

Nutrition profile. ¼ cup:

Calories, 169; fat, 7.1 g (0.7 g saturated, 4.5 g monounsaturated, 7.3 g polyunsaturated); protein, 4.2 g; carbohydrate, 53.4 g; fiber, 5.2 g; cholesterol, 0 mg; sodium, 120 mg.
Omega-3s: ALA, 1.0 g; EPA, none; DHA, none.
Omega-6: 2.3 g.
Ratio of omega-6 to omega-3: 2.3.

Breads and Spreads

Multigrain Flaxseed Bread

One 8-inch round (12 slices)

Flaxseeds lend a healthy dose of alpha-linolenic acid and a beautiful speckled appearance to this bread. When baking breads with flaxseeds, it's common to add a little extra yeast to help the dense bread to rise.

3 teaspoons dry yeast
1 cup warm water (100 degrees to 110 degrees)
3 tablespoons honey or brown sugar
1½ cups all-purpose flour
⅓ cup whole wheat flour
⅓ cup oats
⅓ cup flaxseed meal (ground flaxseeds)
2 tablespoons wheat germ
1½ teaspoons salt
2 tablespoons flaxseeds
canola oil

Sprinkle the yeast into a large mixing bowl, add the water, and let stand for 5 minutes to activate the yeast. Add the honey.

Combine 1¼ cups of all-purpose flour, the whole wheat flour, oats, the flaxseed meal, the wheat germ, and the salt in a small bowl. Add the flour mixture to the yeast mixture, and stir until a soft dough forms (the dough will feel tacky). Turn the dough out on a lightly floured surface and knead until it is smooth and elastic, about 5 to 6 minutes.

Place 2 tablespoons of flaxseeds in a coffee grinder, and pulse a few times to crush them lightly. Sprinkle the seeds on a lightly floured surface, and knead into the dough. Continue to add enough of the remaining flour, 1 tablespoon at a time, to prevent the dough from sticking to your hands.

Place the dough in a lightly oiled bowl, and cover with a kitchen towel or plastic wrap. Let rise in a warm place for about 1½ hours, or until doubled in bulk. Punch the dough down lightly, and shape it into a 6-inch round loaf. Place the dough on a baking sheet lightly brushed with canola oil. Cover and let rise in a warm place for 1 hour, or until doubled in size.

Preheat the oven to 375 degrees. Bake for 30 minutes, or until the bread sounds hollow when tapped. Remove from the pan, and cool on a wire rack.

Cooking tip. This bread works best as a free-form loaf. Left in a loaf pan, it rises poorly and has a flat rather than rounded top.

Nutrition profile. 1 slice:

Calories, 118; fat, 1.8 g (0.2 g saturated, 0.1 g monounsaturated, 1.1 g polyunsaturated); protein, 3.9 g; carbohydrate, 22.6 g; fiber, 2.3 g; cholesterol, 0 mg; sodium, 294 mg.
Omega-3s: ALA, 0.9 g; EPA, none; DHA, none.
Omega-6: 0.2 g.
Ratio of omega-6 to omega-3: 0.2.

Apricot-Flaxseed Tea Bread

ONE 8-INCH LOAF (12 SLICES)

This dense quick bread contains three stellar sources of alpha-linolenic acid: flaxseed meal, omega-3-rich eggs, and canola oil. Apple butter, which adds spice to this recipe, can be found in the supermarket in the jam and jelly aisle.

¾ cup apple cider or apple juice
1 cup chopped dried apricots (about 6 ounces)
⅓ cup brown sugar
¼ cup canola oil
1 tablespoon apple butter
2 omega-3-rich eggs
⅓ cup raisins
1 cup all-purpose flour
½ cup flaxseed meal (ground flaxseeds)
1½ teaspoons baking soda
½ teaspoon salt

Preheat the oven to 350 degrees.

Bring the apple cider to a boil in a small saucepan. Remove from the heat, and stir in the apricots. Let stand 10 minutes. Place ½ cup of the apricot mixture in a small food processor or blender and puree. Combine the puree, brown sugar, oil, apple butter, and eggs; stir well with a whisk. Stir in the raisins and remaining apricots.

Combine the flour, flaxseed meal, baking soda, and salt in a large bowl. Make a well in the center of the mixture, and add the apricot mixture, stirring just until moist. Spoon the batter into an 8- by 4-inch loaf pan lightly coated with canola oil. Bake for 40 to 45 minutes or until a wooden pick inserted in the center comes out clean.

Cool 10 minutes, and remove the bread from the pan. Cool completely on a wire rack.

Cooking tip. Any combination of dried fruit will work for this quick bread. Make sure to rehydrate the dried fruit with a hot liquid such as apple cider or another fruit juice.

Nutrition profile. 1 slice:

Calories, 205; fat, 8.7 g (0.9 g saturated, 3.6 g monounsaturated, 3.6 g polyunsaturated); protein, 4.5 g; carbohydrate, 28.5 g; fiber, 2.8 g; cholesterol, 37 mg; sodium, 279 mg.
Omega-3s: ALA, 2.5 g; EPA, none; DHA, 0.01 g.
Omega-6: 1.5 g.
Ratio of omega-6 to omega-3: 0.6.

Focaccia with Anchovies and Walnuts

16 SERVINGS

Focaccia is an Italian flatbread similar to pizza dough that's traditionally made with lots of olive oil. Here we've switched to canola oil and topped it as they do in parts of northern Italy with a strongly flavored pair; anchovies and walnuts. The nuts provide alpha-linolenic acid, and the anchovies deliver a small helping of EPA and DHA.

1 package active dry yeast (2¼ teaspoons)
1½ cups warm water
1½ teaspoons kosher or sea salt, divided
4 tablespoons canola oil, divided
3¼ to 3½ cups all-purpose flour, divided
2 cloves garlic, finely minced
¼ teaspoon freshly ground pepper
one 2-ounce can anchovy fillets in oil, drained and cut into
    large pieces
⅓ cup coarsely chopped walnuts

Combine the yeast and ½ cup of the warm water in a large bowl. Let stand 5 minutes to activate the yeast. Stir in the remaining water, 1 teaspoon of the salt, 2 tablespoons of the oil, and 3¼ cups of flour. Mix well.

Turn the dough out onto a floured surface, and knead with the remaining ¼ cup of flour, adding 1 tablespoon at a time until the dough is smooth and soft, about 8 minutes. Place the dough in a lightly oiled bowl, and cover with a kitchen towel or plastic wrap. Let rise about 1½ hours, or until doubled in bulk.

Lightly oil a 9- by 13-inch pan or large baking sheet with canola oil. Gently stretch the dough to form a rectangle. (The dough will spring back as you try to stretch it. You may need to let it rest for 5 to 10 minutes to complete the stretching.) Cover and allow to rise until doubled in bulk, about 1 hour.

Preheat the oven to 425 degrees.

Press your fingers into the dough to form indentations or dimples. Combine the garlic and remaining canola oil, and brush the dough lightly with it. Sprinkle the dough evenly with the remaining ½ teaspoon salt and pepper. Sprinkle the anchovies and nuts evenly over the top, and press them in gently with your fingers. Bake for 30 to 35 minutes, or until golden.

Cooking tip. You can omit the anchovies, if desired, and add other toppings, such as sliced onions, olives, and part-skim mozzarella cheese. For a shortcut, use frozen bread dough. Follow the package instructions for rising, and shape and cover with the toppings as directed above. The texture will be slightly different, but the health benefits will remain the same since the omega-3s are all in the topping.

Nutrition profile. 1 piece, about ⅟₁₆ of the rectangle:

Calories, 153; fat, 5.5 g (0.5 g saturated, 2.5 g monounsaturated, 2.8 g polyunsaturated); protein, 4.1 g; carbohydrate, 21.6 g; fiber, 1 g; cholesterol, 0 mg; sodium, 281 mg.
Omega-3s: ALA, 0.8 g; EPA, 0.01 g; DHA, 0.03 g.
Omega-6: 1.6 g.
Ratio of omega-6 to omega-3: 1.9.

Lemon-Herb Flax Butter

½ CUP OR 24 TEASPOONS

Enhancing butter with fresh herbs and other flavorings is nothing new. Here we've lowered the saturated fat of butter and increased the alpha-linolenic acid content by mixing it with equal parts of flaxseed oil. (Flaxseed oil has roughly 7 grams of alpha-linolenic acid per tablespoon.) The end product is a soft spread, much like tub margarine. Use it over steamed vegetables, or omit the lemon and try it on mashed potatoes.

4 tablespoons butter
4 tablespoons flaxseed oil
1 teaspoon butter
1 tablespoon finely chopped shallots
1 tablespoon minced fresh herbs (parsley, basil, dill, or thyme)
¼ teaspoon fresh grated lemon rind

Soften the 4 tablespoons of butter to room temperature in a small bowl. Add the oil and stir with a whisk until smooth. Set aside.

Heat the 1 teaspoon of butter in a small skillet over medium heat. Add the shallots and cook for 2 to 3 minutes, or until softened. Remove from the pan and let cool. Stir the shallots, herbs, and lemon rind into the butter-flax mixture. Cover and chill for at least 1 hour.

Cooking tip. You can make a plain batch of flax butter by mixing equal parts of softened butter and flaxseed oil. Flavored butters keep 3 to 5 days in the refrigerator. Plain flax butter keeps for several weeks.

Nutrition profile. 1 teaspoon:

Calories, 39; fat, 4.4 g (1.5 g saturated, 1.0 g monounsaturated, 1.7 g polyunsaturated); protein, 0 g; carbohydrate, 0.1 g; fiber, 0 g; cholesterol, 6 mg; sodium, 21 mg.
Omega-3s: ALA, 1.2 g; EPA, none; DHA, none.
Omega-6: 0.3 g.
Ratio of omega-6 to omega-3: 0.3.

Smoked Mackerel Spread

1½ CUPS

Traditionally, smoked fish spread or paté is made with butter, cream, or even cream cheese. Here, chickpeas are used to give the spread body without the saturated fat. Mackerel provides a hefty dose of omega-3s, but smoked trout is a great substitute for the mackerel.

½ pound smoked mackerel or trout fillets, skinned
½ cup cooked chickpeas
¼ cup coarsely chopped celery
2 tablespoons coarsely chopped red onion
1½ tablespoons fresh lemon juice
1 tablespoon canola or flaxseed oil
½ teaspoon hot sauce
¾ teaspoon salt

Break the mackerel fillets into pieces. Place the fish and the remaining ingredients in a food processor and process until smooth, scraping down the sides of the processor bowl as needed.

Serve the spread with toasted slices of French bread, pita bread, or whole grain crackers.

Cooking tip. To save time, use canned chickpeas, but be sure to adjust the salt to taste since canned chickpeas are processed with salt.

Nutrition profile. 1 tablespoon:

Calories, 29; fat, 1.5 g (0.2 g saturated, 0.4 g monounsaturated, 0.8 g polyunsaturated); protein, 2.8 g; carbohydrate, 1.1 g; fiber, 0.2 g; cholesterol, 7 mg; sodium, 106 mg.
Omega-3s: ALA, 0.3 g; EPA, 0.1 g; DHA, 0.2 g.
Omega-6: 0.2 g.
Ratio of omega-6 to omega-3: 0.3.

Breakfast

Oatmeal-Flax Pancakes

6 SERVINGS (12 PANCAKES)

Ground flaxseeds, which are high in alpha-linolenic acid, give a subtle nutty undertone to these easy-to-fix hot cakes. Because the hot cakes cook quickly, it's fine to use flaxseed oil in this application.

1½ cups fat-free or reduced-fat buttermilk
½ cup quick-cooking oats (not instant)
1 omega-3-rich egg
2 tablespoons flaxseed or canola oil
1 cup all-purpose flour
¼ cup flaxseed meal (ground flaxseeds)
3 tablespoons white sugar or brown sugar
½ teaspoon salt
1 teaspoon cinnamon
½ teaspoon baking soda
¼ teaspoon baking powder
canola oil (optional)

Combine the buttermilk and oats in a small bowl, and let stand 10 minutes so that the oats absorb the liquid. Stir in the egg and the oil.

Combine the flour, flaxseed meal, sugar, salt, cinnamon, baking soda, and baking powder in a large bowl, and stir well. Add the oat mixture to the flour mixture, stirring until smooth.

Spoon about ¼ cup of the batter for each pancake onto a nonstick griddle or skillet brushed lightly with canola oil, and cook over medium to medium-high heat. Do not crowd the pancakes. Turn the pancakes when their tops are covered with bubbles and the edges look cooked (about 2 to 3 minutes). Finish cooking until the second side is brown, about 1 to 2 minutes.

Cooking tip. Sprinkle some finely chopped walnuts into the batter just before cooking to add an extra dose of alpha-linolenic acid and a more pronounced nut flavor.

Nutrition profile. 2 pancakes:

Calories, 267; fat, 9.1 g (1.0 g saturated, 3.8 g monounsaturated, 3.6 g polyunsaturated); protein, 8.5 g; carbohydrate, 42.3 g; fiber, 2 g; cholesterol, 39 mg; iron, 2.1 mg; sodium, 400 mg.
Omega-3s: ALA, 1.97 g; EPA, 0.01 g; DHA, 0.02 g.
Omega-6: 1.4 g.
Ratio of omega-6 to omega-3: 0.7.

Make-Ahead Breakfast Casserole

8 SERVINGS

This casserole can be made the night before and then baked when you get up in the morning. Each serving contains one omega-3-rich egg and very little saturated fat since the sausage is made with turkey and the cottage cheese is low in fat.

3 teaspoons canola oil, divided
½ cup finely chopped green pepper
¼ cup chopped red onion
1 teaspoon salt, divided

½ teaspoon coarsely ground black pepper, divided
½ cup 1 percent cottage cheese
½ teaspoon dried basil
2½ cups skim milk
8 omega-3-rich eggs, lightly beaten
2 tablespoons chopped fresh parsley
one 12-ounce loaf stale or toasted French bread, cut into
    1-inch cubes
one 3-ounce link of spicy Italian turkey sausage, cooked and
    crumbled

Heat 2 teaspoons canola oil in a large skillet. Add the green pepper and onion, and sauté for 5 minutes. Stir in ½ teaspoon salt and ¼ teaspoon ground pepper, and continue cooking for 4 to 5 more minutes, or until the onion and green pepper begin to soften.

Place the cottage cheese, the remaining ½ teaspoon salt, the remaining ¼ teaspoon pepper, and basil in a food processor or blender, and process until smooth. In a large bowl, combine the cottage cheese, milk, onion and pepper mixture, eggs, and parsley. Stir with a whisk until well blended.

Arrange half of the bread cubes in a single layer in an 11- by 7-inch baking dish brushed lightly with 1 teaspoon canola oil. Spoon half of the egg mixture evenly over the bread slices. Sprinkle the sausage evenly over the layer. Repeat the procedure with the remaining bread and egg mixture. Cover and chill overnight.

Preheat the oven to 350 degrees when ready to bake. Uncover the casserole, and let it stand at room temperature for 10 minutes. Bake for 40 to 45 minutes, or until set.

Nutrition profile. 3½-by-2¾-inch portion:

Calories, 281; fat, 11.4 g (2.9 g saturated, 4.4 g monounsaturated, 3.6 g polyunsaturated); protein, 28.1 g; carbohydrate, 34 g; fiber, 1.6 g; cholesterol, 227 mg; sodium, 714 mg.
Omega-3s: ALA, 0.5 g; EPA, 0.05 g; DHA, 0.15 g.
Omega-6: 1.3 g.
Ratio of omega-6 to omega-3: 1.9.

Ordering Omega-3-Rich Foods

Although many large supermarkets and health-food stores carry the omega 3-rich-foods called for in our recipes, there may be times when a particular ingredient is difficult to find. Here is a rundown of companies that package everything from flax to eggs to buffalo and sell their wares via the Internet or mail order.

Flaxseed and Flaxseed Meal

Storage tip. Flaxseed, because of its fragile omega-3 oil content, needs to be kept in a cool, dark place. Whole seeds will keep for many months at room temperature. Ground seeds (flax meal) should be kept in the refrigerator.

Making flaxseed meal. Grind flaxseeds in a clean coffee grinder until they are pulverized, about 5 to 10 seconds, to make your own meal. One-half cup flaxseeds produces about three-quarters cup of meal.

SOURCES

Bob's Red Mill
3209 Southeast International Way
Milwaukie, OR 97222
1-800-553-2258
www.bobsredmill.com

King Arthur Flour
P. O. Box 876
Norwich, CT 05055
1-800-827-6836
www.home.kingarthurflour.com

Flaxseed Oil

This delicate oil is seldom found in supermarkets, but is available in gourmet food shops and health-food stores. There are many brands on the market. Flavors can vary from brand to brand, from a nutty taste to mildly bitter.

Storage tip. Like the seeds, flaxseed oil can spoil quickly. After opening, store oil in the refrigerator and use it up quickly.

Cooking tip. Do not fry foods with flaxseed oil. Heating this oil at the temperatures used to sauté or fry foods results in the destruction of the omega-3 chemical structure. However, flaxseed oil can be used in breads, muffins, and pancakes because the temperature within these foods is not high enough to destroy the omega-3 fatty acid.

SOURCES

Barlean's Organic Oils
4936 Lake Terrel Road
Ferndale, WA 98248
1-800-445-FLAX

Flax Liquid Gold, Flax Lignan Gold
Health from the Sun
P.O. Box 840
Sunapee, NH 03782
e-mail: efa@hfts.com

Spectrum Essentials
Petaluma, CA 94952
1-800-995-2705
www.spectrumnaturals.com

Game Meats (Venison, Buffalo)

Although not many supermarkets deal in wild game meats, good mail-order sources are plentiful. Some offer a variety of game meats; others sell only buffalo products. The omega-3 content of farm-raised game meat, just like farm-raised fish, will vary, depending on what they are fed.

SOURCES

Denver Buffalo Company
(buffalo meat only)
1120 Lincoln Street, Suite 905
Denver, CO 80203
1-800-BUY-BUFF (1-800-289-2833)

Frontier Buffalo
(buffalo meat only)
75 Maiden Lane
New York, NY 10038
(212) 402-5440

MacFarlane Farms
(pheasant and game meat)
2821 South U.S. Highway 51
Janesville, WI 53546
1-800-345-8348
(608) 757-7881
www.pheasant.com

Seattle's Finest Exotic Meats
(all natural, farm-raised game meat)
17532 Aurora Avenue North
Seattle, WA 98133
(206) 546-4922
1-800-680-4375
www.exoticmeats.com

Silver Bison Ranch
(buffalo meat only)
1954 50th Avenue
Baldwin, WI 54001
(715) 684-2811
www.silverbison.com

Virginia's Buffalo Meats, Inc.
(farm-raised game and specialty meats)
P.O. Box 456
Blue Ridge, VA 24064
(540) 977-5976

Omega-3-Rich Eggs

Eggs are not normally high in omega-3 fats, but several manufacturers are boosting the levels of omega-3 fats by altering the diets of laying hens, feeding them grains, flaxseed, and/or fish meal. Be sure to use the yolk of these eggs; the white is fat free.

SOURCES

The Country Hen
(free-roaming, salmonella-free hens fed organic feed; 170
    milligrams omega-3 per egg—with EPA and DHA)
P.O. Box 333
Hubbardston, MA 01452
(508) 928-5414
www.countryhen.com

Eggland's Best
(hens fed a vegetarian diet with no animal fat; 100 milligrams
    omega-3 per egg)
Eggland's Best, Inc.
King of Prussia, PA
1-800-922-3447
www.eggland.com

Gold Circle Farms Eggs
(hens fed an all-natural, vegetarian diet; 150 milligrams
   omega-3 per egg)
Omega Tech, Inc.
4909 Nautilus Court North, Suite 208
Boulder, CO 80301
(303) 381-8100

Pilgrim's Pride EggsPlus
(hens fed a diet of natural grain and flaxseed; 200 milligrams
   omega-3 per egg)
2777 Stemmons Freeway, Suite 850
Dallas, TX 75207
1-800-824-1159

Purslane

Typically in season during the summer months, this green is a common ingredient in Middle Eastern cooking. It can sometimes be found in specialty stores catering to that cuisine, and there is some availability, albeit spotty, from companies that market fresh herbs and greens on the Internet. If you can't find it and have a green thumb, you might consider growing the green yourself. Here are some sources for the seeds.

SOURCES

Seeds of Change
P.O. Box 15700
Santa Fe, NM 87506

Territorial Seed Company
P.O. Box 157
Cottage Grove, OR 97424

Appendix A:
Conventional and Complementary Medications for Treating Mood Disorders

TABLE A-1: Herbal Psychopharmacology

AGENT	INDICATIONS	BENEFITS	DRAWBACKS
St. John's Wort (Hypericum perforatum)	Major depression Dysthymia	Effective in mild-to-moderate depression Few side effects	May be less effective for severe depression All studies flawed Sunburn risk increased Nausea Reports of serotonin syndrome[1] More research required Different brands have different potencies
SAMe (S-adenosylmethionine)	Major depression Dysthymia	Appears effective Few side effects May help arthritis	Very expensive High rate of inducing mania Effectiveness demonstrated only at very high dosages May increase risk for heart attacks by raising homocysteine levels More research required Different brands have varying stability of compound
Omega-3 Fatty Acids (Fish oil and flaxseed oil)	Bipolar disorder Major depression Dysthymia Schizophrenia Attention deficit hyperactivity disorder? Alzheimer's dementia?	Effective across a wide range of psychiatric and medical disorders Well tolerated Many other health benefits An essential nutrient	High dosages sometimes required Minimum effective dosage unknown Occasional gastrointestinal side effects at high doses Inferior brands may have a fishy aftertaste Flaxseed oil may precipitate mania More research required
Inositol	Major depression Dysthymia Panic disorder Obsessive compulsive disorder To reverse lithium side effects	Appears effective Well tolerated	Expensive High doses often required Difficult to find powder form (dosage is too high to easily use capsules) Inconvenient May precipitate mania More research required

Kava Kava (Piper methysticum)	Anxiety Insomnia	Effective	Excessive drowsiness Intoxication possible Nausea May cause sexual side effects Dry skin
Valerian root (Valeriana officinalis)	Anxiety Insomnia	Effective	Excessive drowsiness Intoxication possible
Melatonin	Insomnia Jet lag Shift work	Effective in mild cases	May be ineffective in severe cases Inflated clinical claims
Ginkgo biloba	Sexual dysfunction due to SSRIs Dementia	Mildly effective	Rare cases of excessive bleeding at high dosages Different brands have different potencies
Antioxidant vitamins Vitamin E 600 to 1200 IUs per day Vitamin C 1,000 mg per day	To prevent or reverse tardive dyskinesia, a serious side effect of antipsychotic medications To boost the safety and effectiveness of omega-3 fatty acids	No known side effects Many other health benefits Essential nutrients	Very limited data exist More research required
L-carnitine	Weight gain due to Depakote (divalproex sodium)	No known side effects L-carnitine is found naturally in the liver and assists in fat metabolism	Anecdotal data only More research required
Acidophilus	Medication-induced diarrhea	Appears effective No known side effects Acidophilus is a beneficial bacteria found naturally in yogurt	Anecdotal data only More research required
Gingerroot	Nausea from medication Dizziness from medication (e.g., BuSpar)	Appears effective No known side effects Found in many Asian recipes	Anecdotal data only More research required Different brands have different potencies

© 1999 Andrew L. Stoll, M.D., Psychopharmacology Research Laboratory, McLean Hospital, Harvard Medical School.

Many of these selections are derived from anecdotal or open-label data only.

These treatments are considered "dietary supplements," and the quality, efficacy and toxicity have not been systematically evaluated or approved by the FDA.

"Natural" does not imply safety; these are pharmacological agents with potential adverse affects.

1. Serotonin syndrome is an uncommon but serious reaction to drugs or compounds with strong effects on the neurotransmitter serotonin. The risk of developing serotonin syndrome is increased if two or more compounds with serotonin effects are mixed together. St. John's wort appears to have effects on serotonin, similar to antidepressant drugs like Prozac, an SSRI (selective serotonin reuptake inhibitor). Although some practitioners recommend mixing St. John's wort with SSRIs to enhance the antidepressant effects or to reduce side effects of the SSRIs, there have been a few reports of serotonin syndrome with this mixture. This chart is for informational use only. Contact your health-care provider for questions and concerns.

TABLE A-2: Commonly Used Mood Stabilizers

TRADE NAME (GENERIC NAME)	INDICATIONS	SIDE EFFECTS	BENEFITS	DRAWBACKS
Depakote* (valproate)	Bipolar disorder Epilepsy or seizures Migraine headaches	Nausea Drowsiness Weight gain Hair loss (rare) Tremor Birth defects Platelet dysfunction (rare) Pancreatitis (rare)	Proven effective in mania Rapidly effective in mania Works better than lithium for different subtypes of bipolar disorder (rapid cycling, mixed mania, and others) Relatively nontoxic Long history of use in epilepsy Good for lithium-unresponsive cases	Side effects Weight gain very common Controversy over whether valproate causes polycystic ovary syndrome; blood tests required
Lithobid, Eskalith CR (lithium carbonate*)	Bipolar disorder	Nausea and/or diarrhea Tremors Increased urination Increased thirst Weight gain Acne Worsening of psoriasis Drowsiness Cognitive dulling Low thyroid function (uncommon) Long-term kidney damage (rare)	Proven effective in mania Proven effective for long-term use 50 years of use The only mood stabilizer with proven antisuicide effects	Side effects Toxicity Not very effective in certain subtypes of bipolar disorder (rapid cycling, mixed mania, and others) Often fatal in overdose Stigma of receiving lithium Blood tests required
Tegretol (carbamazepine)	Bipolar disorder Epilepsy or seizures Chronic pain	Dizziness Drowsiness Double vision May lower disease-fighting white blood cells Skin rashes	Proven effective in mania Good for lithium-unresponsive cases Little or no weight gain	Side effects Toxicity May lose effectiveness over the long term Frequently causes drug interactions

Drug	Uses	Side effects	Benefits	Comments
Calan SR (verapamil)	Bipolar disorder High blood pressure Migraine headaches	Low blood pressure Constipation Sexual side effects	Probably effective in mania Relatively nontoxic No weight gain No blood tests required	Side effects More data required
Lamictal (lamotrigine)	Bipolar disorder Unipolar major depression Epilepsy or seizures	Skin rash (common) Potentially deadly skin reaction: Stevens-Johnson Syndrome (rare)	Strong antidepressant effects Mood stabilizing No weight gain No drowsiness No cognitive effects No blood tests required	To avoid skin reactions, lamotrigine must be started at a very low dosage and increased very slowly. Thus, it may take several months to reach an effective dosage. Valproate will raise lamotrigine blood levels, initially increasing risk of skin rash.
Neurontin (gabapentin)	Bipolar disorder Epilepsy or seizures Anxiety disorders Insomnia Chronic pain	Drowsiness Difficulty with balance and walking (uncommon)	Relieves insomnia No weight gain (at low dosage) Relieves anxiety Nontoxic, even in overdose No drug interactions	Lacks data supporting effectiveness in bipolar disorder Excessive drowsiness Short duration of action which means 2 to 4 divided doses must be taken through the day at high dose range Risk of falls in the elderly due to sedative effects
Omega-3 fatty acids (from fish oil)	Bipolar disorder Unipolar major depression Attention deficit-hyperactivity disorder Heart disease Rheumatoid arthritis Crohn's disease	Nausea and/or diarrhea at high doses	Strong antidepressant effects Mood stabilizing No weight gain No drowsiness No cognitive effects No blood tests required Nontoxic, even in overdose Many other health benefits High-concentration and tasteless supplement available	Some cases of mania with flaxseed oil Not covered by most insurance plans

*Only lithium and Depakote are FDA approved for bipolar disorder.

TABLE A-3: Antidepressant Treatment Guide

Trade Name (generic name)	Drug Class	Indications for Use **	Side-Effect Guide							Comments
			Drowsiness	Weight Gain	Sexual Side Effects	Dry Mouth, Constipation	Nausea	Drug Interaction Risk		
Pamelor* (nortriptyline)	Tricyclic anti-depressant	Depression Panic disorder Generalized anxiety Neuropathic pain	+++	+++	+	+++	–	–	Highly effective More than 40 years of use Often lethal in overdose EKG and laboratory monitoring often required
Parnate (tranylcypromine)	Monoamine oxidase (MAO) inhibitors	Depression Panic disorder Social anxiety disorder	+	+	+	+	–	++++	The most effective antidepressants Certain foods are restricted Dangerous drug interactions Insomnia Low blood pressure when standing up
Nardil (phenelzine)			++	+++	++	++	–	++++	
Desyrel (trazodone)	Serotonin receptor blocker	Insomnia (low doses) Depression (high doses)	++++	–	–	–	+	–	Daytime drowsiness common at higher dosages Rare, unremitting penile erection

Drug	Class	Indications							Notes
Wellbutrin SR (bupropion SR)	Norepinephrine and dopamine reuptake inhibitor	Depression Smoking cessation Attention deficit–hyperactivity disorder	–	–	–		+	–	Safe and effective A "first-line" anti-depressant One of the few antidepressants that does not cause weight gain or sexual side effects Identical to Zyban (the smoking cessation drug) Slight seizure risk if used incorrectly or in patients with epilepsy or bulimia
Prozac (fluoxetine)	Selective serotonin reuptake inhibitor (SSRI)	Depression Panic disorder Generalized anxiety Obsessive–compulsive disorder Bulimia	+	++	+++	–	++	+++	Very safe and effective A "first-line" anti-depressant Sexual side effects common and include low sex drive and delayed or inhibited orgasm

TABLE A-3: Antidepressant Treatment Guide (continued)

Trade Name (generic name)	Drug Class	Indications for Use **	Side-Effect Guide						Comments
			Drowsiness	Weight Gain	Sexual Side Effects	Dry Mouth, Constipation	Nausea	Drug Interaction Risk	
Zoloft (sertraline)	Selective serotonin reuptake inhibitor (SSRI)	Depression Panic disorder Generalized anxiety Obsessive-compulsive disorder Bulimia	-	++	+++	-	++	+	Very safe and effective A "first-line" anti-depressant Sexual side effects common and include low sex drive and delayed or inhibited orgasm
Paxil (paroxetine)	Selective serotonin reuptake inhibitor (SSRI)	Depression Panic disorder Generalized anxiety Obsessive-compulsive disorder Social phobia Bulimia	+	+++	+++	+	++	+++	Very safe and effective A "first-line" anti-depressant Sexual side effects common and include low sex drive and delayed or inhibited orgasm
Luvox (fluvoxamine)	Selective serotonin reuptake inhibitor (SSRI)	Depression Panic disorder Generalized anxiety Obsessive-compulsive disorder	+	++	++	-	++	++	Very safe and effective A "first-line" anti-depressant Sexual side effects common and include low sex drive and delayed or inhibited orgasm

Drug	Class	Indications						Comments
Celexa (citalopram)	Selective serotonin reuptake inhibitor (SSRI)	Depression Panic disorder Generalized anxiety Obsessive-compulsive disorder	+	+	++	-	++	-	Very safe and effective A "first-line" antidepressant Sexual side effects possibly less common and include low sex drive and delayed or inhibited orgasm
Effexor XR (venlafaxine XR)	Serotonin and norepinephrine reuptake inhibitor	Depression Panic disorder Generalized anxiety Obsessive-compulsive disorder	+	++	+++	+	+++	-	Very safe and effective A "first-line" antidepressant Sexual side effects common and include low sex drive and delayed or inhibited orgasm Occasional induction of high blood pressure Blood pressure monitoring required

TABLE A-3: Antidepressant Treatment Guide (continued)

Trade Name (generic name)	Drug Class	Indications for Use **	Side-Effect Guide						Comments
			Drowsiness	Weight Gain	Sexual Side Effects	Dry Mouth, Constipation	Nausea	Drug Interaction Risk	
Serzone (nefazodone)	Serotonin receptor blocker and SSRI action	Depression Generalized anxiety	+++	-	-	+	++	++	Very safe and effective A "first-line" anti-depressant More difficult to use initially but is one of the few antidepressants that does not cause weight gain or sexual side effects Improved sleep
Remeron (mirtazapine)	Serotonin- and norepinephrine releaser and serotonin receptor blocker	Depression Generalized anxiety	++++	+++	-	-	-	-	Very safe and effective A "first-line" anti-depressant More difficult to use initially but is one of the few antidepressants that does not cause sexual side effects Improved sleep Stimulates appetite

© 1995–2000 Andrew L. Stoll, M.D., Psychopharmacology Research Laboratory, McLean Hospital and Harvard Medical School.

* There are other approved tricyclic antidepressants.

** Indications for use does not imply FDA approval.

TABLE A-4: High-Quality Fish Oil Products

NAME	COMPANY	CHARACTERISTICS	FOR INFORMATION OR TO ORDER
Omega-Brite	Omega Natural Science Waltham, MA	90 percent omega-3 fatty acids 7-to-1 ratio of EPA to DHA 500 mg capsules Nitrogen encapsulation	1-888-43-OMEGA *www.omegabrite. com*
Pro-Omega	Nordic Naturals Aptos, CA	50 percent omega-3 fatty acids 1.4-to-1 ratio of EPA to DHA 500 mg capsules	1-888-662-2544 *www.nordicnaturals. com*
Trader Darwin's Hi Potency Omega-3 EPA	Trader Joe's South Pasadena, CA	50 percent omega-3 fatty acids 1.5-to-1 ratio of EPA to DHA 1000 mg capsules	1-626-441-1177 *www.traderjoes.com*
Fish Body Oils 1000	GNC Pittsburgh, PA	30 percent omega-3 fatty acids 1.5-to-1 ratio of EPA to DHA 1000 mg capsules	1-888-462-2548 *www.gnc.com*
Nature's Bounty EPA fish oil	Nature's Bounty Manufacturing Corp. Long Island, NY	30 percent omega-3 fatty acids 1.5-to-1 ratio of EPA to DHA 1000 mg capsules	1-516-567-9500 *www.natures bounty. com*

Appendix B: References

Key to Journal Abbreviations

Acta Chem Scand:	*Acta Chemica Scandinavica*
Am J Clin Nutr:	*American Journal of Clinical Nutrition*
Am J Epidemiol:	*American Journal of Epidemiology*
Am J Human Biol:	*American Journal of Human Biology*
Am J Obstet Gynecol:	*American Journal of Obstetrics and Gynecology*
Am J Psychiatry:	*American Journal of Psychiatry*
Ann N Y Acad Sci:	*Annals of the New York Academy of Sciences*
Ann Rheum Dis:	*Annals of the Rheumatic Diseases*
Arch Gen Psychiatry:	*Archives of General Psychiatry*
Arch Intern Med:	*Archives of Internal Medicine*
Biol Psychiatry:	*Biological Psychiatry*
Biomed & Pharmacother:	*Biomedicine and Pharmacotherapy*
BMJ:	*British Medical Journal*
Br J Nutr:	*British Journal of Nutrition*
Br J Obste Gynaecol:	*British Journal of Obstetrics and Gynaecology*
Comp Ther:	*Comprehensive Therapy*
Dig Dis Sci:	*Digestive Diseases and Sciences*
Early Hum Dev:	*Early Human Development*
Eur Heart J:	*European Heart Journal*
Eur J Clin Nutr:	*European Journal of Clinical Nutrition*
Eur J Obstet Gynecol Reprod Biol:	*European Journal of Obstetrics, Gynecology and Reproductive Biology*
Eur Respir J:	*European Respiratory Journal*

FASEB J:	*Federation of American Societies for Experimental Biology Journal*
Int J Biochem:	*International Journal of Biochemistry*
J Aff Disorders:	*Journal of Affective Disorders*
J Am Coll Nutr:	*Journal of the American College of Nutrition*
J Biol Chem:	*Journal of Biological Chemistry*
J Chromatogr A:	*Journal of Chromatography A*
J Clin Invest:	*Journal of Clinical Investigation*
J Clin Pharmacol:	*Journal of Clinical Pharmacology*
J Lab Clin Med:	*Journal of Laboratory and Clinical Medicine*
J Lipid Res:	*Journal of Lipid Research*
J Neurochem:	*Journal of Neurochemistry*
J Psychiatr Neurosci:	*Journal of Psychiatry and Neuroscience*
J Rheumatol:	*Journal of Rheumatology*
JAMA:	*Journal of the American Medical Association*
Life Sci:	*Life Sciences*
Med J Aust:	*Medical Journal of Australia*
N Engl J Med:	*New England Journal of Medicine*
Neurosci:	*Neuroscience*
Neurosci Lett:	*Neuroscience Letters*
NeuroToxicol:	*Neurotoxicology*
Nutr Cancer:	*Nutrition and Cancer*
Nutr Rev:	*Nutrition Review*
Perspect Biol Med:	*Perspectives in Biology and Medicine*
Philos Trans R Soc Lond B Biol Sci:	*Philosophical Transactions of the Royal Society of London, Series B, Biological Sciences*
Physiol Behav:	*Physiology and Behavior*
Prog Lipid Res:	*Progress in Lipid Research*
Proc Natl Acad Sci USA:	*Proceedings of the National Academy of Sciences, USA*
Prog Neuro-Psychopharmacol Biol Psychiatry:	*Progress in Neuro-Psychopharmacology and Biological Psychiatry*
Prostaglandins Leukot Essent Fatty Acids:	*Prostaglandins, Leukotrienes and Essential Fatty Acids*
Psychosom Med:	*Psychosomatic Medicine*
Schizophr Res:	*Schizophrenia Research*
Semin Perinatol:	*Seminars in Perinatology*
Semin Thromb Hemost:	*Seminars in Thrombosis and Hemostasis*
World Rev Nutr Diet:	*World Review of Nutrition and Dietetics (Basel)*

Chapter 1: Nature's Mood Enhancers

D. Benton, "Fatty acid intake and cognition in healthy volunteers," presented at the NIH workshop on omega-3 fatty acids and psychiatric disorders, September 2–3, 1998.

J. M. Bourre et al., "Function of dietary polyunsaturated fatty acids in the nervous system," *Prostaglandins Leukot Essent Fatty Acids*, 1993;48:5–15.

F. K. Goodwin and K. R. Jamison, *Manic Depressive Illness* (New York: Oxford University Press, 1990).

J. R. Hibbeln and N. Salem, "Dietary polyunsaturated fats and depression: when cholesterol does not satisfy," *Am J Clin Nutr* 1995;62:1–9.

J. R. Hibbeln, "Fish consumption and major depression," *The Lancet* 1998;351:1213.

J. R. Hibbeln, "Long-chain polyunsaturated fatty acids in depression and related conditions," in *Phospholipid Spectrum Disorder*, M. Peet, I. Glen, and D. Horrobin, eds. (Lancashire, England: Marius Press, 1999), pp. 195–210.

K. R. Jamison, "Manic-depressive illness and creativity," *Scientific American*, February 1995, pp. 62–67.

A. Leaf and P. C. Weber, "A new era for science in nutrition," *Am J Clin Nutr* 1987;45:1048–53.

D. O. Rudin, "The dominant diseases of modernized societies as omega-3 essential fatty acid deficiency syndrome: substrate beriberi," *Medical Hypotheses* 1982;8:17–47.

L. J. Stevens et al., "Omega-3 fatty acids in boys with behavior, learning, and health problems," *Physiol Behav* 1996;59:915–20.

A. L. Stoll and E. Severus, "Mood stabilizers: shared mechanisms of action at postsynaptic signal transduction and kindling processes," *Harvard Review of Psychiatry* 1996;4:77–89.

A. L. Stoll et al., "Omega-3 fatty acids in bipolar disorder: A preliminary double-blind, placebo-controlled trial," *Arch Gen Psychiatry* 1999;56:407–12.

Chapter 2: The Fat of Life

R. C. Atkins, *Dr. Atkins' New Diet Revolution* (New York: Avon Books, 1999).

P. G. Barton and F. D. Gunstone, "Hydrocarbon chain packing and molecular motion in phospholipid bilayers formed from unsaturated lecithins," *J Biol Chem* 1975;250:4470–76.

S. Bergstrom and J. Sjovall, "The isolation of prostaglandin," *Acta Chem Scand* 1957;11:1086.

J. M. Bourre et al., "Function of dietary polyunsaturated fatty acids in the nervous system," *Prostaglandins Leukot Essent Fatty Acids* 1993;48:5–15.

G. O. Burr and M. M. Burr, "A new deficiency disease produced by the rigid exclusion of fat from the diet," *J Biol Chem* 1929;82:345–67.

Z. Cohen, H. A. Norman, and Y. M. Heimer, "Microalgae as a source of omega-3 fatty acids," *World Rev Nutr Diet* 1995;77:1–31.

T. R. Dawber, *The Framingham Study: The Epidemiology of Atherosclerotic Disease* (Cambridge, Mass.: Harvard University Press, 1980).

J. R. Hibbeln, "Fish consumption and major depression," *The Lancet* 1998;351:1213.

R. T. Holman, "Biological activities of and requirements for polyunsaturated acids," *Progress in the Chemistry of Fats and Other Lipids* 1970;9:607–81.

A. Keys, *Seven Countries: A Multivariate Analysis of Diet and Coronary Heart Disease* (Cambridge, Mass.: Harvard University Press, 1980).

W. E. M. Lands, "Biochemistry and physiology of n-3 fatty acids," FASEB J 1992;6:2530–36.

David R. Lide, ed., *Handbook of Chemistry and Physics*, 74th ed. (Cleveland, Ohio: CRC Press, 1998).

S. N. Meydani, "Effect of n-3 polyunsaturated fatty acids on cytokine production and their biologic function," *Nutrition* 1996;12:S8–S14.

"Omega-3 Fatty Acids and the Risk in Adults of Cardiovascular Disease" [FDA prohibits labeling omega-3 rich foods as heart healthy], Federal Register, Vol. 63, No. 119, Monday, June 22, 1998, Rules and Regulations, Department of Health and Human Services, Food and Drug Administration: Food Labeling: Health Claims.

D. Ornish et al., "Can lifestyle changes reverse coronary heart disease? The Lifestyle Heart Trial," *The Lancet* 1990;21;336:129–33.

A. J. Parkinson et al., "Elevated concentrations of plasma ω-3 polyunsaturated fatty acids among Alaskan Eskimos," *Am J Clin Nutr* 1994;59:384–88.

E. G. Perkins and W. J. Visek, eds., *Dietary Fats and Health* (Champaign, Ill.: American Oil Chemists' Society, 1983).

Report of the Dietary Guidelines Advisory Committee on the Dietary Guidelines for Americans in *Dietary Guidelines for Americans 2000* (Washington, D.C.: U.S. Department of Health and Human Services, 2000).

N. Salem, B. Wegher, P. Mena, and R. Uauy, "Arachidonic and docosahexanoic acids are biosynthesized from their 18-carbon precursors in human infants," *Proc Natl Acad Sci USA* 1996;93:49–54.

N. Salem and G. R. Ward, "Are omega-3 fatty acids essential nutrients for mammals?" in *Nutrition and Fitness in Health and Disease*, A. P. Simopoulos, ed. (Basel: Krager, 1993).

A. P. Simopoulos, ed., "Nutrition and Fitness in Health and Disease," *World Rev Nutr Diet* 1993;72:128–47.

A. P. Simopoulos, R. R. Kifer, and R. E. Martin, eds., *Health Effects of Polyunsaturated Fatty Acids in Seafoods* (New York: Academic Press, 1986).

A. P. Simopoulos, A. Leaf, and N. Salem, Jr., "Workshop on the essentiality of and recommended dietary intakes for omega-6 and omega-3 fatty acids," *J Am Coll Nutr* 1999;18:487–89.

H. Sprecher, "Biochemistry of essential fatty acids," *Prog Lipid Res* 1981;20:13–22.

M. E. Stensby, "Nutritional properties of fish oils," *World Rev Nutr Diet* 1969;11:46–105.

D. P. Thomas, "Experiment versus authority [scurvy]," *N Engl J Med* 1969;281:932–34.

T. Yamada et al., "Difference in atherosclerosis between the populations of a fishing and a farming village in Japan," *Ann N Y Acad Sci* 1997 Apr 15;811:412–19.

S. Yehuda and D. I. Mostofsky, eds., *Handbook of Essential Fatty Acid Biology* (Totowa, New Jersey: Humana Press, 1997).

Chapter 3: The Evolution Story

P. Andrews and L. Martin, "Hominoid dietary evolution," *Philos Trans R Soc Lond B Biol Sci* 1991;334:199–209, discussion 209.

C. L. Broadhurst, S. C. Cunnane, and M. A. Crawford, "Rift Valley lake fish and shellfish provided brain-specific nutrition for early *Homo*," *Br J Nutr* 1998;79:3–21.

J. G. Chamberlain, "The possible role of long-chain, omega-3 fatty acids in human brain phylogeny," *Perspect Biol Med* 1996;39:436–45.

M. A. Crawford et al., "Comparative studies on fatty acid composition of wild and domestic meats," *Int J Biochem* 1970;1:295–305.

J. Dyerberg and H. O. Bang, "Hemostatic function and platelet polyunsaturated fatty acids in Eskimos," *The Lancet* 1979;2:433–35.

S. B. Eaton and M. J. Konner, "Paleolithic nutrition revisited: a twelve-year retrospective on its nature and implications," *Eur J Clin Nutr* 1997;51:207–16.

S. B. Eaton et al., "Dietary intake of long-chain polyunsaturated fatty acids during the Paleolithic," *World Rev Nutr Diet* 1998;83: 12–23.

S. B. Eaton, "Humans, lipids and evolution," *Lipids* 1992;27:814–20.

R. A. Foley and P. C. Lee, "Ecology and energetics of encephalization in hominid evolution," *Philos Trans R Soc Lond B Biol Sci* 1991; 334:223–31; discussion 232.

J. L. Guil, M. E. Torija, J. J. Gimenez, and I. Rodriguez, "Identification of fatty acids in edible wild plants by gas chromatography," *J Chromatogr A* 1996;719:229–35.

A. Leaf and P. C. Weber, "A new era for science in nutrition," *Am J Clin Nutr* 1987;45:1048–53.

W. R. Leonard and M. C. Robertson, "Evolutionary perspectives on human nutrition: the influence of brain and body size on diet and metabolism," *Am J Human Biol* 1994;6:77–88.

J. M. Naughton, K. O'Dea, and A. J. Sinclair, "Animal foods in traditional Australian aboriginal diets: polyunsaturated and low in fat," *Lipids* 1986;21:684–90.

A. J. Parkinson et al., "Elevated concentrations of plasma ω-3 polyunsaturated fatty acids among Alaskan Eskimos," *Am J Clin Nutr* 1994;59:384–88.

C. B. Ruff, E. Trinkaus, and T. W., Holliday TW "Body mass and encephalization in Pleistocene *Homo*," *Nature* 1997;387:173–76.

A. P. Simopoulos and N. Salem, Jr., "Purslane: a terrestrial source of omega-3 fatty acids [letter]," *N Engl J Med* 1986;315:833.

A. P. Simopoulos H. A. Norman, J. E. Gillaspy, and J. A. Duke, "Common purslane: a source of omega-3 fatty acids and antioxidants," *J Am Coll Nutr* 1992;11:374–82.

Chapter 4: The Wellness Molecules

Asthma

P. N. Black and S. Sharpe, "Dietary fat and asthma: is there a connection?" *Eur Respir J* 1997;10:6–12.

L. Hodge et al., "Consumption of oily fish and childhood asthma risk," *Med J Aust* 1996;164:137–40.

T. Shimizu, "The future potential of eicosanoids and their inhibitors in paediatric practice," *Drugs* 1998;56:169–76.

Cancer

U. N. Das, "Gamma-linolenic acid, arachidonic acid, and eicosapentanoic acid as potential anticancer drugs," *Nutrition* 1990;6: 429–34.

M. De Longeril et al., "Mediterranean dietary pattern in a randomized trial: prolonged survival and possible reduced cancer rate," *Arch Intern Med* 1998;158:1181–88.

"DHA suppresses human breast cancer tumor growth and metastasis in mice," *Cancer Weekly Plus*, December 28, 1998.

L. Kaizer, N. F. Boyd, V. Kruikov, and D. Tritchler, "Fish consumption and breast cancer risk: an ecological study," *Nutr Cancer* 1989; 12:61–68.

Cardiology

C. M. Albert et al., "Fish consumption and risk of sudden cardiac death," *JAMA* 1998;279:23–28.

A. Ascherio et al., "Dietary intake of marine n-3 fatty acids, fish intake, and the risk of coronary disease among men," *N Engl J Med* 1995;332:977–82.

L. J. Beilin, "Dietary fats, fish, and blood pressure," *Ann N Y Acad Sci* 1993;683:35–45.

C. M. Bellamy, P. M. Schofield, E. B. Faragher, and D. R. Ramsdale, "Can supplementation of diet with omega-3 polyunsaturated fatty acids reduce coronary angioplasty restenosis rate?," *Eur Heart J* 1992;13:1626–31.

G. E. Billman, J. X. Kang, and A. Leaf, "Prevention of sudden cardiac death by dietary pure omega-3 polyunsaturated fatty acids in dogs," *Circulation* 1999;99:2452–57.

H. J. G. Bilo and R. O. B. Gans, "Fish oil: a panacea?," *Biomed & Pharmacother* 1990;44:169–74.

K. H. Bonaa et al., "Effect of eicosapentanoic and docosahexanoic acids on blood pressure in hypertension, a population-based intervention trial from the Tromso study," *New Eng J Med* 1990;322:795–801.

M. H. Bowles et al., "EPA in the prevention of restenosis post PTCA," *Angiology* 1991;42:187–94.

M. L. Burr et al., "Effects of changes in fat, fish, and fibre intakes on death and myocardial reinfarction: diet and reinfarction trial (DART)," *The Lancet* 1989:757–61.

J. G. Chamberlain, "Omega-3 fatty acids and bleeding problems," *Am J Clin Nutr* 1992;55:760.

J. S. Charnock, "Dietary fats and cardiac arrhythmia in primates," *Nutrition* 1994;10:161–169.

W. E. Connor, "Effects of omega-3 fatty acids in hypertriglyceridemic states," *Semin Thromb Hemost* 1988;14:271–84.

W. E. Connor and S. L. Connor, "Should a low-fat, high-carbohydrate diet be recommended for everyone?," *N Engl J Med* 1997;337: 562–63.

M. De Lorgeril, S. Renaud, and N. Mamelle, "Mediterranean alpha-linolenic acid rich diet in secondary prevention of coronary heart disease," *The Lancet* 1994;343:1454–59.

R. Garcia-Closas, L. Serra-Majem, and R. Segura, "Fish consumption, omega-3 fatty acids and the Mediterranean diet," *Eur J Clin Nutr* 1993;47Suppl:S85–S90.

L. A. Harker et al., "Interruption of vascular thrombus formation and vascular lesion formation by dietary n-3 fatty acids in fish oil in non-human primates," *Circulation* 1993;87:1017–29.

M. J. Katan, "Fish and heart disease: what is the real story?," *Nutr Rev* 1995;53:228–30.

P. McKeigue, "Diets for secondary prevention of coronary heart disease: can linolenic acid substitute for oily fish?" *The Lancet* 1994;343:1445–54.

M. C. Morris et al., "Fish consumption and cardiovascular disease in the physicians' health study: a prospective study," *Am J Epidemiol* 1995;142:166–75.

B. A. Mueller, R. L. Talber, C. H. Tegeler, and T. J. Prihoda, "The bleeding time effects of a single dose of aspirin in subjects receiving omega-3 fatty acid dietary supplementation," *J Clin Pharmacol* 1991;31:185–90.

S. S. D. Nair, J. W. Leitch, J. Falconer, and M. Garg, "Prevention of cardiac arrhythmia by dietary (n-3) polyunsaturated fatty acids and their mechanism of action," *J Nutr* 1997;127:383–93.

A. Nordoy et al., "Effects of dietary fat content, saturated fatty acids, and parameters in normal men," *J Lab Clin Med* 1994;123: 914–20.

D. Ornish, "Low-fat diets," *N Engl J Med* 1998;338:127.

D. Ornish et al., "Can lifestyle changes reverse coronary heart disease? The Lifestyle Heart Trial," *The Lancet* 1990;21;336:129–33.

H. S. Pedersen et al., "N-3 fatty acids as a risk factor for haemorrhagic stroke," *The Lancet* 1999;353:812–13.

W. E. Severus, B. Ahrens, and A. L. Stoll, "Omega-3 fatty acids—the missing link?" *Arch Gen Psychiatry* 1999;56:380.

A. P. Simopoulos, "Reply to J. G. Chamberlain," *Am J Clin Nutr* 1992;55:760–61.

A. P. Simopoulos, "The nutritional aspects of hypertension," *Comp Ther* 1999;25:95–100.

A. P. Simopoulos and J. Robinson, *The Omega Diet* (New York: Harper-Collins, 1999).

N. J. Stone, "Fish consumption, fish oil, lipids, and coronary heart disease," *Am J Clin Nutr* 1997;65:1083–86.

V. Vaccarino et al., "Sex-based differences in early mortality after myocardial infarction," *New Eng J Med* 1999;341:217–25.

F. Valagussa et al., "Dietary supplementation with n-3 polyunsaturated fatty acids and vitamin E after myocardial infarction: results of the GISSI-Prevenzione trial," *The Lancet* 1999 Aug 7;354(9177):447–55.

P. M. Waring et al., "Leukemia inhibitory factor: association with intraamniotic infection," *Am J Obstet Gynecol* 1994;171:1345–1341.

Y. F. Xiao et al., "Suppression of voltage-gated L-type Ca2+ currents by polyunsaturated fatty acids in adult and neonatal rat ventricular myocytes," Department of Medicine, Harvard Medical School, Boston, MA 02115, USA. *Proc Natl Acad Sci USA* 1997 Apr 15;94(8): 4182–87.

Gastrointestinal System

A. Belluzzi et al., "Effect of an enteric-coated fish-oil preparation on relapses in Crohn's disease," *N Engl J Med* 1996;334:1557–60.

H. J. Hodgson, "Keeping Crohn's disease quiet" [editorial], *N Engl J Med* 1996;334:1599–1600.

F. Kuroki et al., "Serum n3 polyunsaturated fatty acids are depleted in Crohn's disease," *Dig Dis Sci* 1997;42:1137–41.

E. Ross, "The role of marine fish oils in the treatment of ulcerative colitis," *Nutr Rev* 1993;5:47–49.

Lupus

U. N. Das, "Beneficial effect of eicosapentaenoic and docosahexaenoic acids in the management of systemic lupus erythematosus and its relationship to the cytokine network," *Prostaglandins Leukot Essent Fatty Acids* 1994;51:207–13.

D. R. Robinson et al., "Suppression of autoimmune disease by dietary n-3 fatty acids," *J Lipid Res* 1993;34:1435–44.

A. J. Walton et al., "Dietary fish oil and the severity of symptoms in patients with systemic lupus erythematosus," *Ann Rheum Dis* 1991 Jul;50(7):463–66.

Obesity and Diabetes

R. C. Atkins, *Dr. Atkins' New Diet Revolution* (New York: Avon Books, 1999).

M. Barkman et al., "Effects of fish oil supplementation on glucose and lipid metabolism in NIDDM," *Diabetes* 1989;38:1314–19.

H. Glauber, P. Wallace, K. Griver, and G. Brechtel, "Adverse metabolic effect of omega-3 fatty acids in non-insulin-dependent diabetes mellitus," *Ann Intern Med* 1988;108:663–68.

L. Hodge et al., "Effect of dietary intake of omega-3 and omega-6 fatty acids on severity of asthma in children," *Eur Respir J* 1998;11:361–65.

K. D. Hopkins, "Ways of changing sensitivity to insulin," *The Lancet* 1997;350:341.

J. Luo et al., "Dietary (n-3) polyunsaturated fatty acids improve adipocyte insulin action and glucose metabolism in insulin-resistant rats: relation to membrane fatty acids," *J Nutr* 1996;126:1951–58.

T. H. Malasanos and P. W. Stacpoole, "Biological effects of omega-3 fatty acids in diabetes mellitus," *Diabetes Care* 1991;14:1160–79.

D. Ornish, "Low-fat diets," *N Engl J Med* 1998;338:127.

D. Ornish et al., "Can lifestyle changes reverse coronary heart disease? The Lifestyle Heart Trial," *The Lancet* 1990;21;336:129–33.

A. A. Rivellese et al., "Long-term effects of fish oil on insulin resistance and plasma lipoproteins in NIDDM patients with hypertriglyceridemia," *Diabetes Care* 1996;19:1207–13.

S. K. Saha, H. Ohinata, T. Ohno, and A. Kuroshima, "Thermogenesis and fatty acid composition of brown adipose tissue in rats rendered hyperthyroid and hypothyroid—with special reference to docosahexaenoic acid," *Japanese Journal of Physiology* 1998;48:355–64.

L. H. Storlien et al., "Fish oil prevents insulin resistance induced by high-fat feeding in rats," *Science* 1987;237:885–88.

H. Takeuchi et al., "Diet-induced thermogenesis is lower in rats fed a lard diet than those fed a high oleic acid safflower oil diet or a linseed oil diet," *J Nutr* 1995;125:920–95.

Rheumatoid Arthritis

L. G. Cleland et al., "Clinical and biochemical effects of dietary fish oil supplements in rheumatoid arthritis," *J Rheumatol* 1988;15:1471–75.

J. M. Kremer et al., "Dietary fish oil and olive oil supplementation in patients with rheumatoid arthritis: clinical and immunologic effects," *Arthritis and Rheumatism* 1990;33:810–20.

J. A. Shapiro et al., "Diet and rheumatoid arthritis in women: a possible protective effect of fish consumption," *Epidemiology* 1996;7:256–63.

Chapter 5: Pregnancy and Postpartum Depression

M. D. Al et al., "Biochemical EFA status of mothers and their neonates after normal pregnancy," *Early Hum Dev* 1990;24:239–48.

G. O. Burr and M. M. Burr, "A new deficiency disease produced by the rigid exclusion of fat from the diet," *J Biol Chem* 1929;82:345–67.

P. W. Davidson et al., "Effects of prenatal and postnatal methylmercury exposure from fish consumption on neurodevelopment: outcomes at 66 months of age in the Seychelles Child Development Study," *JAMA* 1998;280:701–7.

J. Farquharson et al., "Infant cerebral cortex phospholipid fatty-acid composition and diet," *The Lancet* 1992;340:810–13.

FDA Response to Request to Add Long-Chain Essential Fatty Acids to Infant Formula, March 4, 1999, Public Health Service, Food and Drug Administration, Washington, D.C. *http://www.verity.fda.gov/search97*

M. M. Foreman-van Drongelen et al., "Essential fatty acid status measured in umbilical vessel walls of infants born after a multiple pregnancy," *Early Hum Dev* 1996;46:205–15.

J. R. Hibbeln, "Long-chain polyunsaturated fatty acids in depression and related conditions," in *Phospholipid Spectrum Disorder*, M. Peet, I. Glen, and D. Horrobin, eds. (Lancashire, England: Marius Press, 1999), pp. 195–210.

G. Hornstra, M. D. Al, A. C. Houwelingen, and M. M. Foreman-van Drongelen, "Essential fatty acids in pregnancy and early human development," *Eur J Obstet Gynecol Reprod Biol* 1995;61:57–62.

M. Kaufman, "Baby formula fight puts fat under fire," *Washington Post*, June 1, 1999, retrieved June 2, 1999 from the World Wide Web: *http://www.washingtonpost.com/wp-srv/health/daily/june99/formula1.htm*

M. Kaufman, "What's in infant formula?" *Washington Post*, June 1, 1999, retrieved June 2, 1999 from the World Wide Web: *http://www.washingtonpost.com/wp-srv/health/feed/health928232263965.htm*

A. Lucas et al., "Breast milk and subsequent intelligence quotient in children born preterm," *The Lancet* 1992;339:261–64.

M. Martinex and I. Mougan, "Fatty acid composition of human brain phospholipids during normal development," *J Neurochem* 1998; 71:2528–33.

J. L. Mills et al., "Prostacyclin and thromboxane changes predating clinical onset of preeclampsia: a multicenter prospective study," *JAMA* 1999;282:356–62.

M. Neuringer, S. Reisbick, and J. Janowsky, "The role of n-3 fatty acids in visual and cognitive development: current evidence and methods of assessment," *J Pediatrics* 1994;125:S39–S49.

S. F. Olsen et al., "Randomised controlled trial of effect of fish-oil supplementation on pregnancy duration," *The Lancet* 1992;339:1003–7.

J. L. Onwude et al., "A randomised double blind placebo controlled trial of fish oil in high risk pregnancy," *Br J Obstet Gynaecol* 1995;102:95–100.

F. A. Oski, "What we eat may determine who we can be," *Nutrition* 1997;13:220–21.

S. J. Otto et al., "Maternal and neonatal essential fatty acid status in phospholipids: an international comparative study," *Eur J Clin Nutr* 1997;51:232–42.

S. J. Otto, A. C. van Houwelingen, A. Badart-Smook, and G. Hornstra, "The postpartum docosahexanoic acid status of lactating and non-lactating mothers," *Lipids* 1999;34:S227.

S. Reddy, T. A. B. Sanders, and O. Obeid, "The influence of maternal vegetarian diet on essential fatty acid status of the newborn," *Eur J Clin Nutr* 1994;48:358–68.

A. L. Richardson et al., "Essential fatty acids in dyslexia: theory, evidence and clinical trials," in *Phospholipid Spectrum Disorder*, M. Peet, I. Glen, and D. Horrobin, eds. (Lancashire, England: Marius Press, 1999), p. 229.

N. Salem, B. Wegher, P. Mena, and R. Uauy, "Arachidonic and docosahexaenoic acids are biosynthesized from their 18-carbon precursors in human infants," *Proc Natl Acad Sci USA* 1996;93:49–54.

D. T. Scott et al., "Formula supplementation with long-chain polyunsaturated fatty acids: are there developmental benefits?," *Pediatrics* 1998;102:e59.

A. P. Simopoulus, "Omega-3 fatty acids in health and disease and in growth and development," *Am J Clin Nutr* 1991;54:438–63.

A. P. Simopoulus, A. Leaf and N. Salem, Jr., "Workshop on the essentiality of and recommended dietary intakes for omega-6 and omega-3 fatty acids," *J Am Coll Nutr* 1999;18:487–89.

R. Uauy et al., "Role of essential fatty acids in the function of the developing nervous system," *Lipids* 1996;31:S167–S176.

R. Uauy and D. R. Hoffman, "Essential fatty acid requirements for normal eye and brain development," *Semin Perinatol* 1991;15:449–55.

R. Uauy, "Are omega-3 fatty acids required for normal eye and brain development in the human?" *J Pediatr Gastroenterol Nutr* 1990;11:296–302.

A. C. van Houwelingen, E. C. Ham, and G. Hornstra, "The female do-cosahexaenoic acid status related to the number of completed pregnancies," *Lipids* 1999;34:S229.

Y. Wang, H. H. Kay, and A. P. Killam, "Decreased levels of polyunsaturated fatty acids in preeclampsia," *Am J Obstet Gynecol* 1991;164:812–18.

S. H. Werkman and S. E. Carlson, "A randomized trial of visual attention of preterm infants fed docosahexanoic acid until nine months," *Lipids* 1996;31:91–97.

P. Willatts et al., "Effect of long-chain polyunsaturated fatty acids in infant formula on problem solving at 10 months of age," *The Lancet* 1998;352:688–91.

A. Yonekubo et al., "Dietary fish oil alters rat milk composition and liver and brain fatty acid composition of fetal and neonatal rats," *J Nutr* 1993;123:1703–8.

E. E. Ziejdner, A. C. van Houwelingen, A. D. M. Kester, and G. Hornstra, "Essential fatty acid status in plasma phospholipids of mother and neonate after multiple pregnancy," *Prostaglandins Leukot Essent Fatty Acids* 1997;56:395–401.

Chapter 6: Fighting Major Depression with Omega-3 Oils

P. B. Adams, S. Lawson, A. Sanigorski, and A. J. Sinclair, "Arachidonic acid to eicosapentaenoic acid ratio in blood correlates positively with clinical symptoms of depression," *Lipids* 1996;31 suppl:S157–S161.

American Psychiatric Association, *Diagnostic and Statistical Manual of Mental Disorders: 4th Ed.* (Washington, D.C.: American Psychiatric Association, 1994).

S. Chalon et al., "Dietary fish oil affects monoaminergic neurotransmission and behavior in rats," *J Nutr* 1998 Dec;128(12):2512–19.

R. Edwards, M. Peet, J. Shay, and D. Horrobin, "Omega-3 polyunsaturated fatty acid levels in the diet and in red blood cell membranes of depressed patients," *J Aff Disorders* 1998;48:149–55.

D. S. Heron, M. Shinitzky, M. Hershkowitz, and D. Samuel, "Lipid fluidity markedly modulates the binding of serotonin to mouse brain membranes," *Proc Natl Acad Sci USA* 1980;77:7463–67.

J. R. Hibbeln and N. Salem, "Dietary polyunsaturated fats and depression: when cholesterol does not satisfy," *Am J Clin Nutr* 1995;62:1–9.

J. R. Hibbeln, "Essential fatty acid status and markers of serotonin neurotransmission in alcoholism and suicide," presented at the NIH workshop on omega-3 fatty acids and psychiatric disorders, September 2 to 3, 1998.

J. R. Hibbeln, "Fish consumption and major depression," *The Lancet* 1998;351:1213.

J. R. Hibbeln, "Long-chain polyunsaturated fatty acids in depression and related conditions," in *Phospholipid Spectrum Disorder*, M. Peet, I. Glen, and D. Horrobin, eds. (Lancashire, England: Marius Press, 1999), pp. 195–210.

K. R. Jamison, *Night Falls Fast* (New York: Alfred A. Knopf, 1999).

G. L. Klerman and M. M. Weissman, "Increasing rates of depression," *JAMA* 1989;261:2229–35.

W. E. M. Lands, "Biochemistry and physiology of n-3 fatty acids," *FASEB J.* 1992;6:2530–36.

C. La Vecchia, F. Lucchini, and F. Levi, "Worldwide trends in suicide mortality, 1955–1989," *Acta Psychiatr Scand* 1994;90:53–64.

M. Maes et al., "Significantly increased expression of T-cell activation markers (interleukin-2 and HLA-DR) in depression: further evidence for an inflammatory process during that illness," *Prog Neuro-Psychopharmacol Biol Psychiatry* 1993;17:241–55.

M. Maes et al., *Acta Psychiatr Scand* 1993;87:160–66.

M. Maes, "Evidence for an immune response in major depression: a review and hypothesis," *Prog Neuro-Psychopharmacol Biol Psychiat* 1995;19:11–38.

M. Maes et al., "Interleukin-2 and interleukin-6 in schizophrenia and mania: effects of neuroleptics and mood stabilizers," *J Psychiatr Res* 1995;29:141–52.

M. Maes et al., "Fatty acid composition in major depression: decreased omega-3 fractions in cholesteryl esters and increased C20:4 omega 6/C20:5 omega 3 ratio in cholesteryl esters and phospholipids," *J Affect Disord* 1996;38:35–46.

M. Maes and R. S. Smith, "Fatty acids, cytokines, and major depression," *Biol Psychiatry* 1998;43:313–14.

M. Maes et al., "Lowered omega-3 polyunsaturated fatty acids in serum phospholipids and cholesteryl esters of depressed patients," *Psychiatry Res* 1999;85:275–91.

S. N. Meydani, "Effect of n-3 polyunsaturated fatty acids on cytokine production and their biologic function," *Nutrition* 1996;12:S8–S14.

The Nobel Prize Internet Archive: *http://www.almaz.com/nobel/medicine/medicine.html*

M. Peet, B. Murphy, J. Shay, and D. Horrobin, "Depletion of omega-3 fatty acid levels in red blood cell membranes of depressive patients," *Biol Psychiatry* 1998;43:315–19.

M. Peet, I. Glen, and D. Horrobin, *Phospholipid Spectrum Disorder in Psychiatry* (Lancashire, England: Marius Press, 1999).

D. O. Rudin, "The major psychoses and neuroses as omega-3 essential fatty acid deficiency syndrome: substrate pellagra," *Biol Psychiatry* 1981;16:837–50.

W. E. Severus, B. Ahrens, and A. L. Stoll, "Omega-3 fatty acids—the missing link?" *Arch Gen Psychiatry* 1999;56:380.

R. S. Smith, "The macrophage theory of depression," *Med Hypotheses* 1991;35:298–306.

S. M. Stahl, "Selecting an antidepressant by using mechanism of action to enhance efficacy and avoid side effects," *J Clin Psychiatry* 1998;59;Suppl 18:23–29.

A. L. Stoll, C. A. Locke, L. B. Marangell, and W. E. Severus, "Omega-3 fatty acids and bipolar disorder: a review," *Prostaglandins, Leukot Essent Fatty Acids* 1999:60;329–37.

W. Styron, *Darkness Visible* (New York: Random House, 1990).

M. M. Weissman et al., "Cross-national epidemiology of major depression and bipolar disorder," *JAMA* 1996;276:293–99.

Chapter 7: Omega-3 and Bipolar Disorder

American Psychiatric Association, *Diagnostic and Statistical Manual of Mental Disorders: 4th Ed.* (Washington, D. C.: American Psychiatric Association, 1994).

American Psychiatric Association, "Workgroup on bipolar disorder: Practice guideline for the treatment of patients with bipolar disorder," *Am J Psychiatry* 1994;151(12):S1–30.

J. R. Calabrese et al., "Fish oils and bipolar disorder: a promising but untested treatment," *Arch Gen Psychiatry* 1999;56:413–16.

M. P. Freeman and A. L. Stoll, "Mood stabilizer combinations: a review of safety and efficacy," *Am J Psychiatry* 1998;155:12–21.

A. J. Gelenberg, "New anticonvulsants in bipolar and other psychiatric disorders," *Biological Therapies in Psychiatry* 1997;20(6):21–24.

E. S. Gershon, J. H. Hamovit, J. J. Guroff, and J. I. Nurnberger, "Birth-cohort changes in manic and depressive disorders in relatives of bipolar and schizoaffective patients," *Arch Gen Psychiatry* 1987;44:314–19.

M. J. Gitlin, J. Swendsen, T. L. Heller, and C. Hammen "Relapse and impairment in bipolar disorder," *Am J Psychiatry* 1995;152:1635–40.

F. K. Goodwin and K. R. Jamison, *Manic-Depressive Illness* (New York: Oxford University Press, 1990).

D. F. Horrobin and C. N. Bennett, "Depression and bipolar disorder: relationships to impaired fatty acid and phospholipid metabolism and to diabetes, cardiovascular disease, immunological abnormalities, cancer, ageing and osteoporosis: possible candidate genes," *Prostaglandins Leukot Essent Fatty Acids* 1999;60:217–34. Review.

M. Maes et al., "Interleukin-2 and interleukin-6 in schizophrenia and mania: effects of neuroleptics and mood stabilizers," *J Psychiatr Res* 1995;29:141–52.

D. O. Rudin, "The major psychoses and neuroses as omega-3 essential fatty acid deficiency syndrome: substrate pellagra," *Biol Psychiatry* 1981;16:837–50.

D. O. Rudin, "The dominant diseases of modernized societies as omega-3 essential fatty acid deficiency syndrome: substrate beriberi," *Medical Hypotheses* 1982;8:17–47.

S. J. Slater et al., "The modulation of protein kinase C activity by membrane lipid bilayer structure," *J Biol Chem* 1994;269:4866–71.

R. I. Sperling et al., "Dietary omega-3 polyunsaturated fatty acids inhibit phosphoinositide formation and chemotaxis in neutrophils," *J Clin Invest* 1993;91:651–60.

A. L. Stoll et al., "Shifts in diagnostic frequencies of schizophrenia and major affective disorders in six North American psychiatric hospitals," *Am J Psychiatry* 1993;150:1668–73.

A. L. Stoll, C. A. Locke, A. Vuckovic, and P. V. Mayer, "Lithium associated cognitive and functional deficits reduced by a switch to divalproex sodium: a case series," *J Clin Psychiatry* 1996;57:356–59.

A. L. Stoll and E. Severus, "Mood stabilizers: shared mechanisms of action at postsynaptic signal transduction and kindling processes," *Harvard Review of Psychiatry* 1996;4:77–89.

A. L. Stoll et al., "Omega-3 fatty acids in bipolar disorder: a preliminary double-blind, placebo-controlled trial," *Arch Gen Psychiatry* 1999;56:407–12.

A. L. Stoll and L. B. Marangell, "Commentary: fish oils and bipolar disorder: a promising but untested treatment," in reply, *Arch Gen Psychiatry* 1999;56:415–16.

S. N. Young, "The use of diet and dietary components in the study of factors controlling affect in humans: a review," *J Psychiatr Neurosci* 1993;18:235–44.

Chapter 8: The Omega-3 Response to Stress and Violence

S. Fainaru, "Volatile mix of pressure faces teens, specialists say," *The Boston Globe*, April 24, 1999, p. A8.

T. Hamazaki et al., "The effect of docosahexaenoic acid on aggression in young adults: a placebo-controlled double-blind study," *J Clin Invest* 1996;97:1129–33.

E. Siegel, "It doesn't take a law to curb violence," *The Boston Globe*, October 22, 1993, pp. 49, 66.

L. J. Stevens et al., "Omega-3 fatty acids in boys with behavior, learning, and health problems," *Physiol Behav* 1996;59:915–20.

Chapter 9: Omega-3 Deficiency and Attention Deficit

American Psychiatric Association, *Diagnostic and Statistical Manual of Mental Disorders: 4th Ed.* (Washington, D.C.: American Psychiatric Association, 1994).

C. Belzung et al., "Alpha-linolenic acid deficiency modifies distractibility but not anxiety and locomotion in rats during aging," *J Nutr* 1998 Sep;128(9):1537–42.

J. Biederman, "Attention-deficit/hyperactivity disorder: a life-span perspective" [Review], *J Clin Psychiatry* 1998;59(Suppl 7):4–16.

J. M. Bourre et al., "The effects of dietary alpha-linolenic acid on the composition of nerve membranes, enzymatic activity, amplitude of electrophysiological parameters, resistance to poisons and performance of learning tasks in rats," *J Nutr* 1989;119:1880–92.

H. Frances, C. Monier, and J. M. Bourre, "Effects of dietary alpha-linolenic acid deficiency on neuromuscular and cognitive functions in mice," *Life Sci* 1995;57:1935–47.

S. Gamoh et al., "Chronic administration of docosahexaenoic acid improves reference memory-related learning ability in young rats," *Neuroscience* 1999;93:237–41.

National Institutes of Health Web site for the NIMH-sponsored Multimodal Treatment Study of Children with ADHD—Questions & Answers regarding ADHD: *http://www.nimh.nih.gov/events/mtaqa.cfm*

L. M. Robison, D. A. Sclar, T. L. Skaer, and R. S. Galin, "National trend in the prevalence of attention-deficit/hyperactivity disorder and the prescribing of methylphenidate among school-age children," *Clin Pediatrics* 1999;38:209–17.

L. J. Stevens et al., "Essential fatty acid metabolism in boys with attention-deficit hyperactivity disorder," *Am J Clin Nutr* 1995; 62:761–68.

L. J. Stevens et al., "Omega-3 fatty acids in boys with behavior, learning, and health problems," *Physiol Behav* 1996;59:915–20.

Chapter 10: Treating Schizophrenia with Omega-3 Oils

J. P. Allard et al., "Lipid peroxidation during n-3 fatty acid and vitamin E supplementation in humans," *Lipids* 1997;32:535–41.

American Psychiatric Association, *Diagnostic and Statistical Manual of Mental Disorders: 4th Ed.* (Washington, D.C.: American Psychiatric Association, 1994).

D. F. Horrobin, A. I. M. Glen, and K. Vaddadi, "The membrane hypothesis of schizophrenia," *Schizophr Res* 1998;30:193–208.

J. D. E. Laugharne, J. E. Mellor, and M. Peet, "Fatty acids and schizophrenia," *Lipids* 1996;31Supple:S163–S165.

S. P. Mahadik and R. E. Scheffer, "Oxidative Injury and Potential Use of Antioxidants in Schizophrenia," *Prostaglandins Leukot Essent Fatty Acids* 1996;55:45–54.

J. E. Mellor and M. Peet, "Double blind placebo controlled trial of omega-3 fatty acids as an adjunct to the treatment of schizophrenia." *Paper presented at the Winter Schizophrenia Workshop*, Davos, Switzerland, Feb 7 to 13, 1998. Submitted for publication.

M. Peet, J. D. E. Laugharne, C. Mellor, and C. N. Ramchand, "Essential fatty acid deficiency in erythrocyte membranes from chronic schizophrenic patients, and the clinical effects of dietary supplementation," *Prostaglandins Leukot Essent Fatty Acids* 1996;55:71–75.

B. K. Puri, R. Steiner, and A. J. Richardson, "Sustained remission of positive and negative symptoms of schizophrenia following treatment with eicosapentanoic acid," *Arch Gen Psychiatry* 1998; 55:188–89.

R. C. Wander, S. H. Su, S. O. Ketchum, and K. E. Rowe, "Alphatocopherol influences in vivo indices of lipid peroxidation in postmenopausal women given fish oil," *J Nutr* 1996;126:643–52.

Chapter 11: Memory and Cognition

B. M. Cohen and G. S. Zubenko, "Aging and the biophysical properties of cell membranes," *Life Sci* 1985;37:1403–9.

S. Delion et al., "Age-related changes in phospholipid fatty acid composition and monoaminergic neurotransmission in the hippocampus of rats fed a balanced or an n-3 polyunsaturated fatty acid-deficient diet," *J Lipid Res* 1997;38:680–89.

D. F. Horrobin, "Loss of delta-6-desaturase activity as a key factor in aging," *Medical Hypotheses* 1981;7:1211–20.

S. Kalmijn, E. J. Feskens, L. J. Launer, and D. Kromhout, "Polyunsaturated fatty acids, antioxidants, and cognitive function in very old men," *Am J Epidemiol* 1997;145:33–41.

M. Okada et al., "The chronic administration of docosahexaenoic acid reduces the spatial cognitive deficit following transient forebrain ischemia in rats," *Neurosci* 1996;71:17–25.

M. Vreugdenhil et al., "Polyunsaturated fatty acids modulate sodium and calcium currents in CA1 neurons," *Proc Natl Acad Sci USA* 1996;93:12559–563.

S. Yehuda and R. L. Carasso, "Modulation of learning, pain thresholds, and thermoregulation in the rat by preparations of free purified alpha-linolenic and linoleic acids: determination of the optimal omega-3-to-omega-6 ratio," *Proc Natl Acad Sci* 1993; 90:10345–349.

C. Young et al., "Cancellation of low-frequency stimulation-induced long-term depression by docosahexaenoic acid in the rat hippocampus," *Neurosci Lett* 1998;247:198–200.

Chapter 12: Psychopharmacology and the Health-Food Store

K. M. Bell, L. Plon, W. E. Bunney, and S. G. Potkin, "S-adenosyl methionine treatment of depression: a controlled clinical trial," *Am J Psychiatry* 1988;145:1110–14.

G. M. Bressa, "S-adenosyl-1-methionine (SAMe) as antidepressant: meta-analysis of clinical studies," *Acta Neurol Scand Suppl* 1994;154: 7–14.

G. L. Cantoni, "Biological methylation; selected aspects," *Ann Rev Biochem* 1975;890:435–51.

M. W. P. Carney, B. K. Toone, and E. H. Reynolds, "S-adenosylmethionine and affective disorder," *Am J Medicine* 1987;104–106.

M. W. P. Carney, T. K. N. Chary, T. Bottiglieri, and E. H. Reynolds, "The switch mechanism and the bipolar/unipolar dichotomy," *Br J Psychiatry* 1989;154:48–51.

J. M. Cott and A. Fugh-Berman, "Is St. John's wort (Hypericum perforatum) an effective antidepressant?" *J Nerv Ment Dis* 1998; 186:500–501.

J. Cott, "Medicinal plants and dietary supplements: sources for innovative treatments or adjuncts: an introduction," *Psychopharm Bulletin* 1995;31(1):131–37.

J. Cott, "Natural product formulations available in Europe for psychotropic indications," *Psychopharm Bulletin* 1996;31(4):745–51.

G. Cowley and A. Underwood, "What is SAMe?," *Newsweek*, July 5, 1999, pp. 46–50.

F. C. Czygan et al. *Herbal Drugs and Phytopharmaceuticals: A Handbook for Practice on a Scientific Basis*, N. G. Bisset and M. Wichtl, eds. (Boca Raton, CRC Press, 1994).

P. A. de Smet and W. A. Nolen, "St. John's Wort as an antidepressant," *British Medical Journal* 1996;313:241–47.

K. R. Downum and E. Rodriguez, "Toxicological action and ecological importance of plant photosensitizers," *J Chem Ecol* 1986;12:823–34.

D. M. Eisenberg et al., "Unconventional medicine in the United States: prevalence, costs, and patterns of use," *New England J Medicine* 1993;328:246–52.

A. Fugh-Berman and J. M. Cott, "Dietary supplements and natural products as psychotherapeutic agents," *Psychosom Med* 1999; 61:712–28.

K. D. Hansgen, J. Vesper, and M. Ploch, "Multicenter double-blind study examining the antidepressant effectiveness of the hypericum extract LI 160," *J Geriatric Psychiatry Neurology* 1994;7(suppl 1):s15–18.

G. Harrer, W. D. Hobner, and H. Podzuweit, "Effectiveness and tolerance of the hypericum extract LI 160 in comparison with imipramine: randomized double-blind study with 135 outpatients," *J Geriatric Psychiatry Neurology* 1994;7(suppl 1):s24–28.

W. D. Hubner, S. Lande, and H. Podzuweit, "Hypericum treatment of mild depression with somatic symptoms," *J Geriatric Psychiatry Neurology* 1994;7(suppl 1):s12–14.

B. L. Kagan, D. L. Sultzer, N. Rosenlicht, and R. H. Gerner, "Oral S-adenosylmethionine in depression: a randomized, double-blind, placebo-controlled trial," *Am J Psychiatry* 1990;147:591–95.

K. Linde et al., "St John's wort for depression—an overview and meta-analysis of randomised clinical trials," *BMJ* 1996;313:253–58.

W. E. G. Muller and R. Rossel, "Effects of hypericum extract on the expression of serotonin receptors," *J Geriatric Psychiatry Neurology* 1994;7(suppl 1):s63–64.

M. T. Murray and J. E. Pizzorno, *Encyclopedia of Natural Medicine* (Rocklin, Calif.: Prima Publishing, 1991), p. 268.

M. T. Murray, "St. John's wort (Hypericum Perforatum)," in *The Healing Power of Herbs* (Rocklin, Calif.: Prima Publishing, 1992).

M. T. Murray, *Natural Alternatives to Prozac* (New York: William Morrow, 1996) pp. 130–39.

C. A. Newall, L. A. Anderson, and J. D. Phillipson, *Herbal Medicines: A Guide for Health-Care Professionals.* (London: The Pharmaceuticals Press, 1996), pp. 250–57.

S. Perovic and W. E. G. Muller, "Pharmacological profile of Hypericum extract: effect on serotonin uptake by postsynaptic receptors," *Arzneimittel-Forschung* 1995;45(11):1145–48.

H. Sommer and G. Harrer. "Placebo-controlled double-blind study examining the effectiveness of a hypericum preparation in 105 mildly depressed patients," *J Geriatric Psychiatry Neurology* 1994;7(suppl 1):s9–11.

O. Suzuki et al., "Inhibition of monoamine oxidase by hypericin," *Planta Medica* 1984;50:272–74.

H. M. Thiede and A. Walper, "Inhibition of MAO and COMT by Hypericum extracts and hypericin," *J Geriatric Psychiatry Neurology* 1994;7(suppl 1):s54–56.

E. U. Vorbach, W. D. Hobner, and K. H. Arnoldt, "Effectiveness and tolerance of the hypericum extract LI 160 in comparison with imipramine: randomized double-blind study with 135 outpatients," *J Geriatric Psychiatry Neurology* 1994;7(suppl 1):s19–23.

H. Wagner and S. Bladt, "Pharmaceutical quality of hypericum extracts," *J Geriatric Psychiatry Neruology* 1994;7:s65–68.

Chapter 13: The Omega-3 Renewal Plan

Z. Cohen, H. A. Norman, and Y. M. Heimer, "Microalgae as a source of omega-3 fatty acids," *World Rev Nutr Diet* 1995;77:1–31.

J. Eritsland, "Safety considerations of polyunsaturated fatty acids," *Am J Clin Nutr* 2000;71(suppl):197S–201S.

T. Ninomiya et al., "Expansion of methylmercury poisoning outside of Minamata: an epidemiological study on chronic methylmercury poisoning outside of Minamata," *Environ Res* 1995 Jul;70(1):47–50.

D. Pauly and V. Christensen, "Primary production required to sustain global fisheries," *Nature* 1995;374:255–57.

T. A. B. Sanders, "Vegetarian diets and children," *Pediatr Clin North Am* 1995;42:955–65.

A. P. Simopoulos, A. Leaf, and N. Salem, Jr., "Workshop on the essentiality of and recommended dietary intakes for omega-6 and omega-3 fatty acids," *J Am Coll Nutr* 1999;18:487–89.

Chapter 14: Understanding Omega-3 Supplements

S. C. Cunnane et al., "Nutritional attributes of traditional flaxseed in healthy young adults," *Am J Clin Nutr* 1995;61:62–68.

E. A. M. de Deckere, O. Korver, P. M. Verschuren, and M. B. Katan, "Health aspects of fish and n-3 polyunsaturated fatty acids from plant and marine origin," *Eur J Clin Nutr* 1998;52:749–53.

J. Eritsland, "Safety considerations of polyunsaturated fatty acids," *Am J Clin Nutr* 2000;71(suppl):197s–201s.

D. Farrell, "Enrichment of hen eggs with n-3 long-chain fatty acids and evaluation of enriched eggs in humans," *Am J Clin Nutr* 1998;68:538–44.

J. A. Foran, B. S. Glenn, and W. Silverman, "Increased fish consumption may be risky," *JAMA* 1989;262:28.

B. P. Grubb, "Hypervitaminosis A following long-term use of high-dose fish oil supplements," *Chest* 1990;97:1260.

D. Kenny, "Adverse effects of fish oil," *Arch Intern Med* 1990;150:1967.

B. A. Mueller, R. L. Talbert, C. H. Tegeler, and T. J. Prihoda, "The bleeding time effects of a single dose of aspirin in subjects receiving omega-3 fatty acids," *J Clin Pharmacol* 1991;31:185–90.

J. R. Sargent and G. J. Tacon, "Development of farmed fish: a nutritionally necessary alternative to meat," *Proc Nutr Soc* 1999;58:377–83.

Mercury in Fish—Fish Consumption Advisories

Charts of specific advisories, Michigan Department of Community Health, retrieved November 8, 1999 from the World Wide Web: *http://www.mdch.state.mi.us/pha/fish/charts.htm#general*

EPA fact sheet update: listing of fish and wildlife advisories, 1999, U.S. Environmental Protection Agency, retrieved November 8, 1999 from the World Wide Web: *http://fish.rti.org*

Fish and wildlife reports results of new fish health program, 1999, Agency of Natural Resources Press Releases, retrieved November 8, 1999 from the World Wide Web: *http://www.state.vt.us/database/PressRel/Detail.CFM?Agency ID=123*

Fish consumption advisories in the great lakes region, retrieved November

8, 1999 from the World Wide Web: *http://iet.msu.edu/regchrt/regstate/mifish.htm*

Health alert, 1997, Vermont Department of Health, retrieved November 8, 1999 from the World Wide Web: *http://www.state.vt.us/health/fish.htm*

How much is safe?, 1999, Mayo Foundation for Medical Education and Research, retrieved August 3, 1999 from the World Wide Web: *http://www.mayohealth.org/mayo/9604/htm/merc_sb.htm*

D. O. Marsh et al., "Fetal methylmercury study in a Peruvian fish-eating population," *NeuroToxicol* 1995;16:717–26.

Mercury—current alerts, Vermont Public Interest Research Group, retrieved November 8, 1999 from the World Wide Web: *http://www.vpirg.org/priorities/mercury.cfm*

Mercury in fish: cause for concern?, 1995, U.S. Food and Drug Administration, retrieved August 3, 1999 from the World Wide Web: *http://www.fda.gov/opacom/catalog/mercury.html*

Mercury in fish: concerns shouldn't dampen your appetite, 1999, Mayo Foundation for Medical Education and Research, retrieved August 3, 1999 from the World Wide Web: *http://www.mayohealth.org/mayo/9604/htm/mercury.htm*

D. C. G. Muir, et al., "Arctic marine ecosystem contamination," *Sci Total Environ* 1992;122:75–134.

NWF urges Congress to address problem of mercury contamination in waters of the United States, 1998, National Wildlife Federation, retrieved August 3, 1999 from the World Wide Web: *http://www.nwf.org/greatlakes/pp/s1915.html#FCA*

Appendix C:
Resources for Patients and Families with Depression and Bipolar Disorder

K. R. Ablow and J. R. DePaulo Jr., *How to Cope with Depression: A Complete Guide for You and Your Family* (New York: McGraw-Hill, 1989).

N. C. Andreasen, *The Broken Brain* (New York: Harper and Row, 1984).

D. Berger and L. Berger, *We Heard the Angels of Madness* (New York: William Morrow, 1991).

P. Duke and G. Hochman, *A Brilliant Madness: Living with Manic-Depressive Illness* (New York: Bantam, 1993).

C. Felix, *All About Omega-3 Oils* (New York: Avery Publishing, 1998).

R. R. Fieve, *Moodswing* (New York: Bantam Books, 1973).

F. Goodwin and K. Jamison, *Manic Depressive Illness* (New York: Oxford University Press, 1990).

K. R. Jamison, *Touched with Fire* (New York: Free Press, 1996).

K. R. Jamison, *An Unquiet Mind* (New York: Random House, 1997).

K. R. Jamison, *Night Falls Fast: Understanding Suicide* (New York: Alfred A. Knopf, 1999).

D. Papolos and J. Papolos, *Overcoming Depression* (New York: Harper & Row, 1988).

D. Papolos and J. Papolos, *The Bipolar Child* (New York: Harper & Row, 2000).

D. Rudin and C. Felix, *Omega-3 Oils: A Practical Guide* (New York: Avery Publishing, 1996).

A. P. Simopoulos and J. Robinson, *The Omega Diet* (New York: HarperCollins, 1999).

W. Styron, *Darkness Visible* (New York: Random House, 1990).

Ask Dr. Andrew Weil Web site: *http://www.pathfinder.com/drweil/ qa–answer*

Index